Praise for the *Voices of* Book Series

"Pure inspiration."

Shape Magazine

"...provides answers to practically anyone wondering 'What now?' ...this worthy collection succeeds very well."

Publishers Weekly

"Hearing others' stories is the most substantial aspect of any support group... It's the universality of the emotions that links these essays and puts the human face on what can be a very scary disease. For all patient health collections."

Library Journal

Other Books by The Healing Project

Voices of Alcoholism
Voices of Alzheimer's
Voices of Autism
Voices of Caregiving
Voices of Breast Cancer
Voices of Lung Cancer
Voices of Multiple Sclerosis

Voices of Bipolar Disorder

The Healing Companion: Stories for Courage, Comfort and Strength

Edited by

The Healing Project

www.thehealingproject.org

"Voices Of" Series Book No. 8

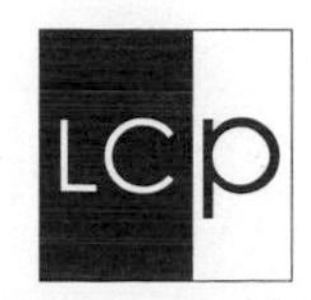

LaChance publishing

LACHANCE PUBLISHING • NEW YORK
www.lachancepublishing.com

ISBN 978-1-934184-07-3

Edited by Richard Day Gore and Juliann Garey

Library of Congress Control Number: 2009935159

Publisher: LaChance Publishing LLC
120 Bond Street
Brooklyn, NY 11217
www.lachancepublishing.com

Distributor: Independent Publishers Group
814 North Franklin Street
Chicago, IL 60610
www.ipgbook.com

This book is available at special discounts for bulk purchases for sales promotions or premiums. Special editions, including personalized covers, excerpts of existing books, and corporate imprints, can be created in large quantities for special needs. For more information, write to LaChance Publishing, 120 Bond Street, New York, NY 11217 or email info@lachancepublishing.com.

Printed on 100% recycled paper.

The journey from beginning to end is not always clear and straightforward. While work on *Voices Of* began just a short time ago, the seeds were planted long ago by beloved sources. This book is dedicated to Jennie, Larry and Denise, who in the face of all things good and bad gave courage and support in excess. But especially to Richard, who taught us by the way he lived his life that anything is possible given enough time, hard work and love.

Contents

The Healing Project

Debra LaChance

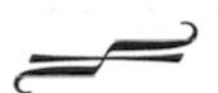

I wanted to ask the people around me, "Would you please raise your hand if you feel as isolated as I do?" Walking the busy streets of Manhattan on a beautiful sunny day, I was surrounded by people but I'd never felt so alone. Just minutes before, my doctors had broken the news to me that I had a particularly aggressive form of breast cancer.

Since moving to New York from a small town in Rhode Island, I'd had my share of ups and downs but had always risen to the challenges that living and working in New York can bring. But on this summer afternoon, I felt as if the world was suddenly rushing past me while I seemed to be moving in slow motion. I was completely alone.

After recovering from the initial shock, I found that one of the first things I almost automatically began to look for, besides doctors, was a sense of connection. I needed to hear from other people who had gone through what I was experiencing, who truly understood what it meant and who might be able to help. I wasn't ready for a regular support group, and with surgery and treatment looming, I simply didn't have the time. But I am an avid reader, and I assumed that finding the personal stories of those who had gone through this ordeal before me would be relatively easy. But there seemed to be a vacuum; almost nothing. Where were the real people to talk to? Where was the literature that wasn't just about the hardcore science of the disease, but about how to cope?

I knew there must be countless others out there who needed to tell their stories—and to hear the stories of others as well. My thoughts kept returning to that walk through Manhattan after I'd heard my diagnosis, and that feeling of terrible loneliness. As sympathetic as friends and loved ones could be, I felt that no one could truly understand this journey except someone who had made it before. I was convinced that getting and giving courage, comfort, and strength were as important as good medical care, and I became determined to help build a community for people like me who were undergoing the terribly isolating experience of dealing with a life-threatening or chronic disease.

Out of this resolve to build a sense of community, The Healing Project was born. The Healing Project's mission is to become a bridge across which people can make those all-important emotional connections. I began to develop The Healing Project as a place where people can contribute funds for research, time for connecting with others, and most of all, a place to share their stories. Since then, The Healing Project has been collecting stories by those touched by illness or diseases for books like this one: books that inspire and inform for the road ahead and impart a sense of community for those caught up in dealing with the moment. These books are meant to be a companion for patients, their friends, and families, an oasis where they can find strength in shared experiences. I don't want anyone to have to feel the way I did the day of my diagnosis when I was walking through the city alone and afraid. There's so much strength in others—you just have to find them.

When you are dealing with disease, you have to be ready to chart a new course, for the rest of your life, no matter what the outcome. And it helps to see that others are busy charting their own courses along with you. That's what these stories are all about. Reading these amazing contributions to the Voices Of series convinces me that I don't really have a uniquely remarkable story at all.

The truth is, everyone does.

Debra LaChance is the creator and founder of The Healing Project.

People diagnosed with life-threatening or chronic, debilitating illnesses face countless physical, emotional, social, spiritual, and financial challenges during their treatment and throughout their lives. The support of family members, friends, and the community is essential to their successful recovery and their quality of life, and access to accurate and current information about their illnesses enables them and their caregivers to make informed decisions about treatment and post-treatment care. Founded in 2005 by Debra LaChance, *The Healing Project* is dedicated to promoting the health and well-being of these individuals, developing resources to enhance their quality of life, and supporting the family members and friends who care for them. For more information about *The Healing Project* and its programs, please visit our website at www.thehealingproject.org.

An Introduction to Bipolar Disorder

Marina Benaur, M.D.

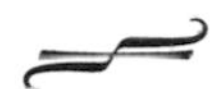

What is Bipolar Disorder?

Our emotional lives are dynamic, and we experience a variety of moods in response to daily events, thoughts and memories that are all part of our inner, subjective experience. At times, we are aware of the particular mood we are experiencing, such as a sensation of pleasure and wellbeing on a calm morning walk, or a sense of irritation and anger after an altercation with a friend. At other times, we may not pay much attention to the positive or negative valence of a particular moment. If experiencing different moods and their fluctuations is a normal, and in some ways an essential part of being human, what, then, constitutes a mood disorder?

Mood disorders are a group of neurobiological illnesses that affect brain function in such a way that the daily experience of moods, their intensity and variability, becomes disrupted. The inner experience of living in the world becomes unreliable; emotions may be too intense, or there may be a lack of feelings that are appropriate to the situation. Moods may change too rapidly or not at all despite the occurrence of significant life events. Mood disorders can be divided into two general categories: *unipolar disorders*, generally referring to the abnormal and sustained decline in mood called *depression*, and *bipolar disorders*, which include syndromes in which mood can either be abnormally low or abnormally elevated, a state known as *mania*.

Since antiquity, mood disorders have been recognized as biological illnesses that tend to run in families. Hippocrates described *melancholia*, or depression, as a syndrome characterized by an "aversion to food, despondency, sleeplessness and irritability." Other Greek physicians saw in some people the tendency to change from the state of depression or melancholia into the agitated state of mania, which was described by Aretaeus as a mood state associated with excessive joy, energy, irritability, agitation, insomnia and erratic behavior, among other symptoms. By the 18th century, the recurrent nature of bipolar mood disorder was captured with the term *folie circulaire*, or circular madness. Emil Kraepelin, the 19th century psychiatrist acknowledged by many as the father of modern scientific psychiatry, developed the term *manic-depressive illness* to describe the disorder, thus capturing the alternating nature of the two mood poles that is its chief characteristic. The modern term for this illness is *Bipolar I* disorder, and we now also recognize that there are less severe forms of the illness that can be described in the aggregate as *bipolar spectrum disorders*.

The Characteristics of Bipolar Disorder

Bipolar I disorder affects approximately 1–2% of the population in the United States. Its usual onset is in late adolescence or young adulthood. The initial mood episode that marks the onset of the illness can be depression or any form of mania, and can occur in response to a stressful life event or it can occur without any clear triggering event. There is no laboratory or neuro-imaging technique that can be used to help diagnose either depression or mania. Therefore, if an abnormal mood state is suspected, an experienced clinician will make the diagnosis based on the symptoms presented and the personal history of the patient. A diagnosis of the disorder can only be made once there is a clear history of at least one manic episode

Depression, or major depressive episode, is a syndrome defined by at least two weeks of sustained low mood, difficulties with sleep and appetite, low energy and concentration, often recurrent guilty feelings, hopelessness and thoughts of death. When untreated, major depressive episodes are dangerous biological conditions that can lead to a severe impairment in daily living, the disruption of work and relationships and can even threaten the patient's life by poor self-care and neglect, and ultimately, by suicide.

Mania, or manic episode, typically develops as a sense of a heightened experience of energy, pleasure, creativity, self-confidence that can progress to a sense of grandiosity, the lack of need for sleep and an overabundance of ideas that makes it difficult to think logically or make rational decisions. Manic episodes are defined as sustained elevated mood for at least a week with prominent excess energy, rapid speech, racing thoughts, distractibility and often impulsive, dangerous, risk-taking behaviors. In the midst of a manic episode, the risks and benefits of a particular decision are not assessed logically, and patients may engage in behaviors that are utterly different from their usual way of life, which might include promiscuity, impulsive overspending, getting into fights and the use of illicit substances. Although the initial symptoms of mania may be pleasurable, its consequences can be severely disruptive to virtually all aspects of one's life, including health, career, and relationships.

Mixed mood episodes, also called *mixed manic episodes*, are perhaps the most disabling, and involve symptoms of both depression and mania occurring concurrently. During a mixed mood episode, a person is dominated by low and negative mood at some moments, while at others he or she might feel irritable, edgy and unable to rest. The person's overall sense of energy is often elevated, but when he or she lacks the ability to direct it productively, it can lead to frustration and agitation, posing the greatest risk for suicide unless promptly treated.

Bipolar I disorder is the most severe form of bipolar spectrum disorders. Its course is characterized by recurrent manic, mixed and depressed states. If someone has had a manic or mixed manic episode without ever having suffered from depression, the diagnosis of Bipolar I disorder is correct, because these severe and disabling mood states are unique to this pattern of the illness. On the other hand, major depressive episodes that occur in the absence of manic or mixed symptoms, even if recurrent, may be part of a unipolar mood disorder pattern that does not warrant a diagnosis of bipolar disorder. It is important to recognize and diagnose bipolar disorder correctly, because specific treatments can be life saving, but it is also important not to over-diagnose the illness and label any emotionally varied or unstable experience a form of bipolar illness. In mood disorders, periods of unusually low or elevated mood are sustained over several days and often weeks, and are also accompanied by sleep, appetite and cognitive changes. Simply being a moody or emotionally intense person does not mean that one has bipolar illness.

Other well-recognized bipolar spectrum illnesses include *Bipolar II disorder* and *Rapid Cycling Bipolar disorder*. With Bipolar II disorder, a person experiences severe episodes of depression alternating with episodes of *hypomania*, a milder form of mania. Hypomanic episodes may last only a few days and do not result in severe disruptions to life, but are still characterized by an unusual increase in energy, a decreased need for sleep and sometimes uncharacteristic irritability. Although the majority of difficulties and disability for patients with Bipolar II disorder stem from recurrent depressions, it is important to elicit the history of hypomania, because treatment for bipolar II disorder is quite different from the treatment of depression alone.

Bipolar disorders vary widely in their severity and presentations. While some people may only have one or two mood episodes in their lifetime and lead relatively unaffected lives, others suffer from multiple episodes, often several times a year. With Rapid Cycling Bipolar disorder, four or more distinct mood episodes occur within a year. This pattern is rare, only seen in about 10% of patients with bipolar disorder, and for reasons that are still unclear seems to predominantly affect women.

The Cause of Bipolar Disorder

Although well described for thousands of years, the underlying neurobiology of bipolar disorder remains elusive and poorly understood. However, since the advent of *neuroimaging* techniques, improved molecular biology and the advance of genetic research, progress has been made in understanding this illness. Bipolar disorder definitely has a genetic component, and tends to cluster in families. First-degree relatives of patients with bipolar disorder are at least twice as likely to be affected by a mood disorder than is the general population. Studies of inheritance patterns in twins has demonstrated a two to four-fold increase in the presence of bipolar disorder in identical versus fraternal twins. While genetic predisposition confers a biological vulnerability, it does not explain why some people with the same genetic risk develop the illness and some do not. After all, identical twins share all of their genetic material, but not all develop the same illness. This pattern is often seen with complex disorders that involve several genes which are malfunctioning together and whose expression is influenced by the environment in which the person develops. Environmental triggers, which can adversely influence biologically vulnerable individuals, are stressful situations such as trauma or loss, events that disturb the sleep/wake cycle, such as studying all night for exams or frequently traveling between time zones, and most certainly, exposure to psychoactive substances such as illicit drugs or steroids.

Some of the most exciting research into the neurobiology of bipolar illness has focused on the deep structures in the brain that regulate *circadian rhythms*, or the sleep-wake cycle of daily activity and rest. Although sleep remains a mysterious frontier in neuroscience, we now know that our brains remain active during sleep in ways that are quite different from wakefulness and that are crucial to survival and health. Most of us also know intuitively from our personal experiences with sleep deprivation or the sense of fatigue that can occur with some depressions that sleep and mood are intimately related. Sleep is markedly disturbed in all phases of bipolar illness, and subtle changes in sleep patterns can be harbingers of mood episodes that are in their earliest stages. Research has shown that genes that are implicated in bipolar disorder may be involved in the regulation of our natural sleep/wake cycle. At least one aspect of abnormal neurobiology may create disordered communication within neural networks that control circadian, or daily, biological rhythms. The involvement of these "time-keeping" neurobiological circuits may be a clue to the cycling, recurrent pattern in bipolar illness that, for some people, has a strong seasonal component. The tendency for manic episodes to appear toward the spring months and depression to worsen during fall and winter months has long been recognized, but only now are we beginning to find clues to the neurobiological basis of these seasonal patterns. Light therapy treatments have been developed to treat depression and can also be used in bipolar disorder based on these principles.

Other research into the cause of the disorder has focused on the neural networks between areas in the brain long known to be involved in the experience of powerful emotions and their regulation. The brain is organized into specialized regions that are in constant communication with each other via multiple overlapping neural networks. One such region, known as the *limbic system*, is a well-defined neural circuit of highly interconnected brain structures including the *amygdala* and *hippocampus* that are intimately involved with the experience and regulation of emotion. Current thinking is that bipolar disorder does not result from an abnormality within any one particular structure in the brain, but rather from a dysregulated pattern of communication between these parts of the limbic system and the *pre-frontal cortex*, that portion of the brain responsible for planning complex cognitive behaviors, personality expression, decision making and moderating correct social behavior.

Neuronal communication involves a variety of substances in the brain called *neurotransmitters*. Abnormalities in neurotransmitter function affect the brain's ability to transmit information and regulate responses to the environment and are involved in the development of mood disorders. The neurotransmitter systems most implicated in bipolar disorder are *norepinephrine*, *serotonin*, *GABA*, *glutamate* and *dopamine*. Our understanding of abnormal neurotransmitter function forms the basis for psychopharmacological treatment of depression and bipolar illness.

Treating Bipolar Disorder

The treatment of bipolar disorder has recently made significant advances, but remains challenging, and, when successful, almost always involves a multifaceted approach that includes more than just medications. It is important to emphasize, however, that bipolar illness is a biologically-based disorder and that the use of medications remains essential in achieving and maintaining recovery.

There are two basic treatment considerations: treatment of the acute mood episode, with the goal of returning to a baseline level of functioning, and maintenance treatment, to prevent future mood episodes and relapse. There is substantial evidence that the more frequent mood episodes occur earlier in the illness, the more frequent and severe future mood episodes will be. This is known as the *kindling hypothesis*, and it argues strongly in favor of early treatment focused on the maintenance of remission and the prevention of future episodes.

Mood stabilizing medications are helpful in ending acute episodes, and are crucial for sustaining recovery. Lithium, which has been used since the 1950s, has a long history as an effective mood stabilizer in bipolar disorder. It has saved countless lives by its unique effect of also improving treatment of depression and preventing suicide more than any other medication developed so far. *Antiepileptic agents*, such as valproic acid (Depakote), carbamazepine (Tegretol) and lamotrigine (Lamictal) are also known to be good stabilizers. Another class of drugs, *atypical antipsychotics* have recently received significant attention for being useful in the treatment of both the acute and the maintenance phases of bipolar illness. Antidepressants can safely be used to treat severe bipolar depression, but exposure to these medications in the absence of adequate mood stabilization can lead to the development of manic or mixed symptoms. Because the treatment of bipolar disorder may sometimes involve the use of several medications at the same time, it is important that an experienced psychiatrist be involved in their selection.

The treatment of bipolar illness can be particularly challenging. Patients often need to be admitted to a hospital for safety monitoring and medication adjustments. In the midst of a manic episode, one can almost never make good judgments and the burden of arranging for the hospitalization and getting vital help usually falls on the family. Being open with one's partner and loved ones about the illness can be extremely helpful in ensuring prompt and appropriate help. Developing a collaborative relationship with a psychiatrist based on mutual trust and respect takes time and work, and it is important to remain in treatment even during the stable times when mood is not disturbed, so as to be in the best position to address even the earliest signs of relapse and prevent a full blown depression or mania.

There are some instances when medications alone are not sufficient to help end an episode of severe depression, mania or mixed state. In those situations *ECT* (electro-convulsive therapy) remains the most effective treatment. ECT is a biological treatment that works by inducing a seizure in the brain under controlled circumstances with an anesthesiologist present throughout the procedure. The effectiveness of ECT is well established in the medical literature; culturally, however, it has often been misrepresented as painful, scary and leading to cognitive difficulties. Though it is true that early ECT treatments did result in more short-term memory deficits than we see today, the bad press has created unnecessary fear of the treatment, which is a life saving option for many people. Modern ECT practice has advanced significantly, and it is a well-tolerated, safe procedure that can quickly relieve the suffering of patients with severe depression or mania that do not improve with medications alone.

In addition to biological treatments for bipolar disorder, *psychotherapy* and *social rhythm therapy* help people adjust to the everyday experience of living with a mood disorder and develop greater control over emotional states. Social rhythm therapy has used what is known about the connection between circadian rhythms and sleep for mood stabilization to develop a system in which a person tracks his or her optimal sleep and activity schedule and develops a routine which creates a more regular day/night schedule to help stabilize mood. Protecting sleep and developing a more organized lifestyle can be as valuable in maintaining recovery as medications. The two approaches work synergistically to help the brain function optimally and avoid triggering a mood episode that can become disabling.

The Case for Hope

Effective treatment of bipolar disorder usually consists of a well-chosen and tolerated medication strategy, psychological support and sometimes psychotherapy in combination with a healthy lifestyle. When understood and adequately treated, bipolar illness can be controlled. Having successfully overcome the initial challenges of aberrant mood states, people can and do lead emotionally rich and varied lives.

Dr. Marina Benaur earned her medical degree from The University of North Carolina–Chapel Hill and went on to complete a combined residency training in neurology and psychiatry at the New York-Presbyterian Hospital of Columbia and Cornell. Board certified in psychiatry, she works in the Columbia University Psychiatry Department as an attending inpatient psychiatrist and also has a private practice in Manhattan. She lives in New York.

Next to Normal: Bipolar Disorder Takes Center Stage

Juliann Garey

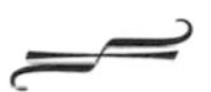

In 1998, while students at New York's prestigious BMI Lehman Engel Musical Theater Workshop, librettist/lyricist Brian Yorkey and composer Tom Kitt chose an odd subject for their first-year final project of creating a ten-minute musical. They wanted to do something… different. Both were close to people who struggled with mental illness of one kind or another, so when Yorkey saw a *Dateline NBC* segment on electroconvulsive therapy, a treatment sometimes used to help those suffering from bipolar disorder, their project was decided and the seed for what eventually became the Tony Award-winning musical *Next to Normal* was planted. It took ten years for the show—which tells the story of the struggles of Diana, a suburban wife and mother with bipolar disorder and the effect it has on her family—to evolve. Ten years—approximately the same length of time it takes for someone with bipolar disorder to receive a proper diagnosis.

Now on Broadway, this bold, brave, uncompromising show with music and lyrics that are at once startlingly truthful and achingly beautiful, is reaching thousands. And slowly but surely, eight shows a week, it is chipping away at the age-old stigma surrounding the disorder. Here, the Tony Award-winning creators and cast of Broadway's *Next to Normal* talk about bringing bipolar disorder center stage.

On the Evolution of the Show

> *I don't need a life that's normal—*
> *that's way too far away*
> *But something...next to normal*
> *would be okay.*
>
> —From "Maybe"

Both Kitt and Yorkey evolved professionally and personally over the period during which they worked on what would become *Next to Normal.* Their perspectives changed, their heroine changed, their show changed. Radically. They were constantly diagnosing and reassessing what treatment would best serve their material.

"We started writing the show," says Kitt, "when I was 24 and Brian was 26. I was a bachelor just out of school. I finished the show at 35, married with a young child. So in terms of personal experience, in terms of the story that we wanted to write and what was going to help illuminate this character's struggle, we came up with different things over time that were affected by our growth. Part of the journey of the show has been focusing it on the family. I think the final version that is now on Broadway, is really the story of this family at its best in this ten year process. We finally, I think, nailed it."

"It was interesting," says Yorkey, "that early on, we were interested in the medical issues and the way the medical establishment works. But it became less and less about that and more and more about the people. Which is to the great credit of our director, Michael Greif, who would often say to us, 'The people are more interesting than the medicine.' At first I didn't know what that meant. I thought, 'It's about the medicine...she's mentally ill.' But then I realized it was about telling this woman's story. The medicine is a part of her story, but it's only part of it. The whole story is the answer to the questions, what is her life and what does it cost her family? David Stone, our producer, asked the right questions early on. He asked, 'Is this show just about the woman or is it about the family?' And we said well, it's about the family. And he said, 'Okay, we need to know more about what this is doing to them.' And a big part of the journey, the evolution of the show, was exploring that issue."

On Making Their Heroine Just a "Normal" Person

I will hold it all together...
We're the perfect loving family...
If they say we're not, then fuck 'em...
The perfect loving family...
I will keep the plates all spinning,
and the world just keeps on spinning,
and I think the house is spinning

—From "Just Another Day"

In large measure, *Next to Normal* is "just" another voice of bipolar disorder because its heroine Diana is "just" a regular person. She is not a famous artist or a rock star or a mad but brilliant astrophysicist. She is a regular person. But that is, in fact, what makes *Next to Normal* so different and so relatable.

"One of the suggestions we got early on," says Yorkey "was that we should make her a poet or a painter so that we could see her creativity get stifled. I think we both felt that she should be a regular person, someone with a life we can all recognize, because I think that so often bipolar and other diseases of the mind tend to get romanticized. There's this idea that a special version of the illness applies to artists and brilliant, creative people, and that these diseases of the mind are torments of their genius. In reality, it is both much more mundane and, I think, much more complex than that. It really became, for us, how Diana negotiates her life and her family and how her family negotiates the illness and that seemed to us to be at once very relatable to so many of us and also really, really dramatic."

"Like Brian said," adds Kitt, "the illness can get lost in the genius of someone and can stand outside the normal person or the average person who lives with this in a much more earthly way their entire life and we wanted this story to reach out to everyone who deals with this and its struggle."

On How No One Behind Next to Normal is Bipolar... Exactly

Perfect for you.
I will be perfect for you.
So you could go crazy,
or I could go crazy
—it's true.
Sometimes life is insane,
but crazy I know I can do...

—From "Perfect For You"

No one on the *Next to Normal* creative team has bipolar disorder, which might seem somewhat controversial. But talk to the cast for a few minutes—scratch the surface just the tiniest bit—and you'll find that no one is all that removed from some type of mental illness.

"My grandmother did a lot of the same stuff Diana does," says Louis Hobson, who plays both the psychopharmacologist and the therapist characters in the show. "My mom saw the show and was like, 'Wow, that was my mom.' And her brother has bipolar disorder. And my mother is on the cusp of battling that as well. She's never been diagnosed, but... so there are a lot of people in my family."

"Yeah," adds Alice Ripley, who won a Tony Award for her performance as Diana, "and I'm no stranger to someone smashing china or shooting a hole through the T.V. with a bullet or smashing the stereo with a hammer. There were several people."

"My youngest sister is obsessive compulsive," chimes in Kyle Dean Massey, who's playing the role of Diana's son Gabe while Aaron Tveit is on leave. "She wore four watches in case they stopped. She's moved past it a lot. But she still has episodes. But it was like, what do I do when she tries to pluck all my eyebrows?"

Jennifer Damiano, nominated for a Tony for the role of teenage daughter Natalie, made her Broadway debut in *Spring Awakening* at age fifteen. She has been fairly quiet during the interview, until now. "My mom locks herself in her room all the time," she says, and shrugs.

No one can accuse this cast of not being able to relate to the material.

"Like everybody," says Kitt, "I am touched in some way by mental illness personally. This is not the story of my life in any way, but we didn't want the show just to be about sensationalized moments of emotion and anger and heartache. Because so much of it is the everyday, the little things that sneak up on you and devastate you. Brian and I both have an understanding about the everyday of it, the moments of the cycle of up and down, when someone is starting to feel better and the devastation when it derails again; it's something that we've all been through. I think we have an understanding of that."

"Neither of us is bipolar," says Yorkey, "but we each have people in our lives, some of whom are friends that we share, who struggle with bipolar or a similar mental disorder. So the idea to try to understand what it's like to have your life ruled by a mind that doesn't always work the way it should was something we wanted to understand in the first place, and then wanted to tell it in a compelling and truthful way."

"At the end of the day," says Kitt, "Brian and I are very passionate about this subject matter and brought everything from our own lives to it."

On the Medicine Behind the Music

Zoloft and Paxil and Buspar and Xanax,
Depakote, Klonapin, Ambien, Prozac,
Ativan calms me when I see the bills—
These are a few of my favorite pills.

—From "Who's Crazy/My Psychopharmacologist and I"

Not only did Kitt and Yorkey do a tremendous amount of research on bipolar disorder, from reading mainstream texts to academic journals, they also had a psychiatrist, a psychologist and various other experts in the field read each and every draft of the show. "They were incredible," says Yorkey. "They'd say, 'Think about this,' or, 'Here's something I've experienced,' or, 'Here's something that we've learned.' So we were able to write this woman very carefully. Her illness is very specific to her, as everybody's is, really. There's no 'one' bipolar. Every person's illness is unique. So all this arguing about 'She has this' or 'She has that…' well, welcome to her life with doctors. One of our consultants offered the opinion that sometimes the best you can do is take a patient's symptoms, put a name to them and try to treat what the symptoms are. Well, it was really interesting to hear a doctor describe the process that way, so I gave that line to the doctor in the show because that's sort of what he's doing. Many people said, 'It's not this, it's not that,' but time and time again, reading books, talking to people, the story was that there was some sort of less obvious predisposition or sensitivity to the illness, and there was a major life event that precipitated the actual illness. I heard that story so many times, and that seemed to make perfect sense in terms of the life Diana had led.

"It was very important to Brian and me every time we took a new pass at it to ask ourselves, 'What in the medicine is not yet there? What do we have to talk about? Who do we need to have read this and give us some expertise about a certain thing?' So we really felt like we had talked about every single issue in this show, and were able to feel comfortable with what's on stage. And of course, everybody has their own personal experience. You can't satisfy every single person who has dealt with this. But hopefully what you can do is give it a fair and adequate setting and treatment so that we're honoring this struggle."

"And," says Yorkey, "give it a face."

"Which, I think, is the other thing," Kitt says. "We were hearing these stories all along the way that were helping us understand more and more what the disease is and what it is to live with it and how to be empathetic with it. And I think that's part of the remarkable journey of the show, that we had people who would share their stories. We would learn things. And many of those things actually ended up in the show and became the stories of these characters."

On the Fear of Bringing Bipolar to Broadway or, the Elephant in the Theater

Make up your mind that you're strong enough.
Make up your mind

—

let the truth be revealed.

—From "Make Up Your Mind"

"For me," says Yorkey, "it was a little bit terrifying, the idea of opening a musical about mental illness on Broadway in the middle of a recession. But at the same time, David Stone, who produced it, was fearless about it. Once he decided to do this show, he has been behind it all the way. He never once told us, 'Oh, the ending needs to be happier.' He never flinched. That gave me a lot of confidence."

"I've already seen how bad it can go on Broadway," says Kitt. "But I stand by this show no matter what happens. I'm proud of it, I'm proud of the subject matter. I believe there's an audience, based on what I've seen, that wants to experience this show. If it doesn't work out, I have no regrets, because in my heart I wanted to bring the show to as wide an audience as I could. So, yes of course, it's scary, but at the end of the day, it would have been scarier not to get the opportunity."

In other words, Yorkey sums it up: "They can kill you but they can't eat you."

"Exactly," says Kitt, "I feel like we're telling the story in a truthful, compelling and honorable way and now what happens, happens. There was a lot of terror for me along the way. But ultimately, on opening night, I was very at peace with it."

And apparently they needn't have worried, because the audience reaction to *Next to Normal* is like nothing anyone in the cast has ever experienced before.

"A lot of people come to this show with their 'lens', their perspective," says Hobson. "I think people who have had a bad experience with therapy will see it differently than those who have had a great experience. A lot of therapists come up to me after the show and 95% of the time it's, 'Thank you so much for your honest portrayal of what we do.' I think therapists see themselves, see their own struggles dealing with, as somebody once said to me, 'a soft science.' I think that's exactly true. It's not something that you can read in a textbook. Every patient is different and every person requires something different."

"People relate to the show, even if they don't know anyone or don't have anyone in their family who has bipolar disorder," says

Robert J. Spencer, who plays Dan, Diana's husband. "The show still resonates with them because of the heart of it and because of the family. Because everyone has an issue with their family and loss. And if you are bipolar or have someone in your family who is bipolar, then it is a beautiful additional piece of therapy to your life, and that's tremendous. It's amazing that it can do that for people and help people. A guy came to the stage door a while back and said, 'Thank you for allowing me to grieve.'"

"I've been on other shows," says Ripley, "and never felt this impact where the audience feels so represented. They want to share it, and it's a remarkable change for them. It's transforming. I've done a lot of shows and have never done a show that felt like a community service. That's what it's supposed to be. It feels quadruply good to do this show… it feels good in so many ways."

On the Ending

We'll find the will to find our way,
knowing that the darkest skies
will someday see the sun.
When our long night is done
there will be light.

—From "There Will Be Light"

"I think one of our big hopes for the show," says Yorkey, "is that it will help people to talk about the 'elephant in the room.' One of the big things we did between the Second Stage production and the Broadway production was to rewrite the lyrics to the last song, which was called 'Let There Be Light.' At first, the lyrics were sort of general and vague, but it's such a stirring song that I wanted to rewrite it so that we could keep the song and end the show on a note that's not necessarily optimistic, but definitely has hope to it. So we sat down last summer and thought about what we wanted people to walk away with. The answer was that we wanted people to walk away with this notion that there is no guarantee that things are going to get better and that there are no promises and no easy endings. But there is hope in the struggle, like when Diana says: 'You don't have to be happy at all to be happy you're alive.' And also that the struggle and the pain are part of the whole package, not that that is a particularly profound thought, but after having gone through this, we felt like you had to leave with some notion that it was worth spending these two hours here. And for us, if this experience can lead people to open up their own lives a little bit and shed a little light on it rather than keeping these things secret, rather than just trying to repress what's going on, that would be a worthwhile end.

Next to Normal is currently playing at the Booth Theater on Broadway. For more information and to hear music from the show please visit www.nexttonormal.com.

Acknowledgments

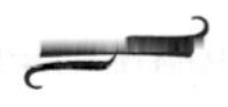

This book would not have been possible without the selfless dedication of many people giving freely of their valuable time and expertise. We'd particularly like to thank Dr. Marina Benaur for her extraordinary and invaluable expertise, and the many, many people who submitted their stories to us, for their courage, their generosity and their humanity.

PART ONE

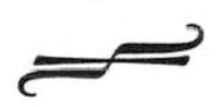

"...depression took my soul and all my self-worth..."

"...fireworks of thoughts were exploding in my brain..."

"...no one can imagine *how it feels*."

Buried Under Water

H. Rachelle Graham

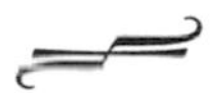

I am at the bottom of a dark ocean with a hundred pounds of concrete on top of my body. My friends and family are snorkeling nearby. I can hear them call out to me, but I cannot see them. They tell me, "The plants and fishes are so pretty and the water feels so warm." I feel nothing but ice cold water and heavy concrete. I cannot move my arms and legs to join them. I am drowning. I cannot breathe. I feel dead. This, for me, is depression.

Mania is even worse. It is as if I am locked inside a bare room, unable to sit still. The nurses wait on guard outside my door, afraid I will hurt myself, more afraid I will get out and hurt them. My thoughts are speeding and my limbs are out of control "Help me," I scream to the nurses. As soon as they come in, I dash like the Energizer Bunny to the exit. At the door, I throw a pitcher of apple juice at one nurse and scratch the other one until she bleeds. The emergency intercom blares that there's a dangerous person on the loose. Two security guards grab me and throw me back into the tiny room. And my hell begins again.

My bipolar started when I was in elementary school. I went to school in a depressed state and spent the majority of my time feeling worthless and inadequate. I never talked to any of the other kids; I thought I was below them. Then I would go home and drive my mother to exhaustion with my constant outbursts of talking, jumping and crying. I was the third daughter of four and the only one who was not allowed to have more than one cookie at a time. If I did, my mania would increase and I would run around until I crashed.

From elementary to high school, I spent my half hour lunches hiding in girls' locker rooms and bathrooms. I hated myself and thought everyone else hated me. I developed verbal and writing skills so late that my mother thought I was autistic. I screamed or flinched when I was touched by anyone.

College and the real world hit me even harder. I struggled and ended up dropping out. I got a job at a credit union from which I was soon fired for leaving every few minutes to go the bathroom or roam around. I simply could not sit still or focus on the work.

My illness literally became a life or death matter when I swallowed an entire bottle of an anti-psychotic drug I was taking to suppress the voices I was hearing and my suicidal thoughts. My body recovered from the overdose, but my mind never did. I was transferred to the University of Neuropsychiatry Hospital in Salt Lake City where I was given Prozac, Ativan and Seroquel and sent home a week later.

The next two years were a living hell. Depression took my soul and all my self-worth. I was so worn out I couldn't bathe. I hated my body. When I went out in public I thought everyone was staring at me with disgust. I believed I would only feel better if I were dead. So I overdosed again. I took a bottle of Tylenol P.M. and then went to work out at Jordan Valley Aquatic Center. I hoped to die in the pool.

I was discharged a week later. The doctor said the electroshock had improved my mood, and it was true. The next year was tough, but I didn't try to hurt myself. I got a job at a local newspaper and that really helped to bolster my mood, so much, in fact, that a year later, I decided I didn't need to take medications anymore. Big mistake, but I hated the side effects, including weight gain and constant dry mouth. I went off them cold turkey and immediately started suffering from huge mood swings. I was sent again to hospital and my doctor started me back on my medication and ECT treatments. I had fifty-five ECT treatments before my mood improved. I went to daily group and individual therapy sessions as well.

> "My thoughts are speeding and my limbs are out of control 'Help me,' I scream to the nurses."

I was then transferred to a longer term hospital a few miles away. There I met an older doctor who wore a silver earring. He always had a wide grin on his face, so I nicknamed him Happy Doc. He seemed to care deeply about all his patients and he took over administering my ECT treatments. I looked forward to every visit with him, and when I saw him I felt a little relief from my depression. At first, I refused to get out of bed in the morning but soon I was locked out of my room and forced to spend a month doing simple activities like crafts, watching T.V., listening to music and participating in group therapy discussions. I eventually started to enjoy myself, and the ECT and drugs began to work their magic once again. I actually started to smile and jump out of bed in the morning, eager to begin a new day.

When my family came to visit, my mom had huge bags under her eyes. I felt so guilty for causing her stress. She had started on antidepressants for the first time in her life because of me. And my older sister worked my guilt. I think she did it so I would stop hurting myself. It worked. I started trying much harder and as a result, Happy Doc discharged me a month later, cutting my ECT treatments to once every other week.

After I got out of the hospital, I began a strict individual and group therapy treatment regimen. One I joined was dialectical behavior therapy, or DBT. This group was extremely helpful in controlling my suicidal impulses and helping me learn other ways to cope with my problems. For example, instead of pulling out a razor to cut myself, I would go for a walk. These choices seem obvious but they made all the difference. Make enough choices correctly and your life becomes much easier to live.

I do try to make the right choices. Every day I take my required medication and use my DBT skills. There are still times I want to hang myself or stay in bed all day, but I ignore these impulses and force myself to leave the house. I have a service dog that I bring everywhere. She is my best friend and a wonderful listener. My family is supportive of my illness and does not blame me for my problems.

I have been out of the hospital for seven years. Bipolar is never easy and I am still learning how to deal with it. The more I fight, the easier it becomes. Therapy has taught me how to love myself and be proud of my accomplishments. I went back to school and finished a Bachelor's degree in journalism. I currently work for a large community paper and I look forward to getting up every day. I don't have the terrible dreams of being buried under concrete, under water. My family and friends don't swim past me; instead we enjoy life together. I can finally see that clear crystal water and feel its warmth. If things start getting rough, I get help from loved ones and mental health professionals. I am alive, again.

H. Rachelle Graham received a Bachelor's degree in journalism and is currently working on a second degree in English at the University of Utah. She has worked for local newspapers, such as *The Salt Lake Tribune*, and *Magna Times* and has had articles published in magazines including *True Love* and *True Story*.

Sui Generous

Juliann Garey

Today my incoming psychopharmacologist (Outgoing Doc is abandoning me for warmer, sunnier, more cheerful climes) let slip that he thinks I'm harboring the "suicide gene." Yes, apparently there is one.

On what does he base this somewhat alarming piece of information, which I of course choose to take—and frankly, who wouldn't—as a death sentence? Admittedly, his evidence is purely anecdotal. But let's start with the fact that he's a big gun in the bipolar world, that he's really smart and that he's got lots of experience. All of that may be vague, but it wins him points nonetheless. Also, he finds my family and me scientifically interesting—at least enough to take me on as a patient. Apparently not always a given with Dr. Incoming. So, more points. Then there's the interesting bit of trivia, borne out by the people who study these things—or, more accurately, the people who are studied—that violent suicides run in families, and that people with violent suicidal ideations (i.e. gun, window/roof, razor vs. some less self-destructive mode of self-destruction like, for example, sleeping pills) are much more likely to have the gene.

Finally there's the fact that there have been four suicides in my family within two generations. My father shot himself and three of his uncles committed suicide—at least one with a gun. There are those in my family who maintain that my great uncle's death was a tragic accident, that his gun went off erroneously. In his mouth. With no one around for miles. So clearly, an accident. Also, they say, one of the two remaining suicides doesn't count because he was really old.

For obvious reasons, I have always been very anti-firearm. But I have an unhealthy fascination with sharp, shiny objects, and most recently, on one bleak winter afternoon, I found myself standing on the top of our couch in front of an open window, sobbing.

Why didn't I jump? That's easy: I don't want to die. But in my most desperate moments I believe I would do, will do, anything to stop the suffocating, all consuming, excruciating misery and panic. And in those moments/hours/days/weeks I cannot fathom the possibility that it might stop on its own. In those moments, it is keeping myself from jumping that is hard. A week ago I was one frosty breath away from the same irrevocable action my father took. The one I'm sure he would have lived to regret. If he had lived.

"I believe I would do anything to stop the suffocating, all consuming, excruciating misery and panic."

I wish I didn't know about the suicide gene. There are lots of things I wish I didn't know. For example, that rapid cycling bipolar disorder, the kind I have, is harder to treat and has a poorer prognosis than other kinds. Or that in all likelihood my hippocampus is shrinking. I wish I could say that's really just a euphemism intended to mean that my ass is getting smaller. No such luck. It means I'm getting dull—cognitively speaking. Socially I'm still the sparkling wonder I always was—a marginally reclusive socio-phobe who works from home. But the brain thing is troubling. It was one of my best features. Now, on most days, holding a thought in my head is like trying to hold water in one hand. The hippocampus is in charge of things like the consolidation of new memories, emotions, navigation, and spatial orientation. Fabulous.

Crazy was a given, but clumsy and stupid? And lost? Well, let's not even go there. Apparently I'd never find my way back.

Outgoing Doctor says when I'm "stable" (a phrase I'm beginning to equate with *when the messiah comes…*), all these faculties will come back to me. Incoming guy says, not so much. The changes are real and permanent. But, he adds, subtle. So, not to worry. Not to worry? As in *light-bulb's-out-in-the-bathroom* not to worry? Or more like *maybe-I-should-start-wearing-a-medic-alert-bracelet-so-that-if-I-get-lost-and-can't-remember-my-own-address-or-name-a-nice-person-will-take-me-home* not to worry? Because there's a big difference.

I take a lot of drugs. These days, none of them seems to do much. But lithium has anti-suicidal properties. Both Dr. Outgoing and Dr. Incoming have told me this: "You need to stay on it," they added, "don't worry about the dose." But one always worries about the dose with lithium because there's a fine line between the therapeutic dose and the toxic one. Too little and it does nothing—except apparently keep you from ending it all—too much and suddenly you're walking into walls, shaking like you've got the DTs and sounding like an idiot. If you ignore all that, there's coma and death. Which sort of undermines the whole point of the drug.

I'm good about taking my lithium. I don't want to die. Those ten minutes on the windowsill were enough to prove to me, to mark me profoundly and indelibly, to make me realize that suicide is not about having a plan. It is not about wanting to get out and away. It is about impulse control. Having and losing it. For only as long as it takes to make the leap or pull the trigger. Not long at all. Sometimes my biggest fear is that the sheer exhaustion of trying to keep it from happening is enough to make it happen.

So I take my lithium. Every fucking day.

Unfortunately, apparently my kidneys don't like it. My internist has sent me to a nephrologist, a kidney doctor. He's been pushing me to do this for almost a year because he suspects I have kidney damage, early stage. From ten years of lithium use. For the last few years, my creatinine levels have been high. That's what they measure to see how well your kidneys are working. My internist, who has known me since before I was diagnosed as bipolar, says my levels shouldn't be so high. And neither should my blood pressure. Both Drs. In and Out have said not to worry about it. They are more concerned with the suicide gene.

I like the nephrologist. She is not afraid of my bipolar disorder. She is not the least bit awkward. She also says she will do everything she can to not take away the lithium. But she doesn't like my creatinine levels. She orders a kidney ultrasound and 24-hour urine collection and blood test to measure creatinine output over the course of a whole day. I will come back in 10 days. Then we will see what's what.

I believe this is what they call a Hobson's choice. Kidney failure or suicide. Or, suicide by kidney failure.

The problem is, I want to live.

At the end of our last appointment, Dr. Outgoing gave me a hug. "Don't lose hope," he said. "There is an answer. There is always an answer. Sometimes you just have to be creative."

Then he told me to call him when I get suicidal.

When, not if.

When.

As if he had looked at me under a microscope and saw me parading around in my genes.

Juliann Garey is a novelist, journalist, screenwriter and Associate Editor at LaChance Publishing. She lives in New York City with her husband and her two children.

Saturday

Lisa Rusczyk

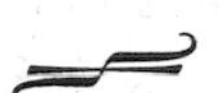

My boyfriend wakes me up at 8 A.M. I don't want to get up and go to his son's ball game. It's going to rain. I didn't sleep well. My boyfriend and I had a fight over my not liking *Donnie Darko*, one of his favorite movies, and he slept on the couch. Our fights are passionate but pointless most of the time.

The main reason I don't want to go to the game is that I think his son hates me. My boyfriend repeatedly tries to explain to me that he's only five, that he likes me, that it's all in my head. I realize that I do need to make an effort. I love this man, I love the boy. I don't want to screw up anything. I don't perceive things the way others do, I know that. I'm bipolar. I climb out of bed and into his arms and thank him for talking sense into me.

Halfway to the ball game we find out it's canceled because of the weather. I'm feeling pretty good because the boy giggled when I was talking to the windshield wipers. "Can't see!" when the rain covered the windshield. "Thank you!" when the boyfriend turned the wipers on for a single swish.

We've been talking about getting a fourth cat. I say, "Since we're out, want to go to the pet store?"

The boyfriend says that's a good idea and the boy thinks so, too. We hit up the only two pet stores in town but they have no kittens. We get a newspaper and make a few calls answering ads for free kittens, but nobody answers. I leave messages. I say I want to take us all out to eat while we wait for return calls. I only have $100 in my account to last until the end of the month because I haven't been feeling well enough to work, but this is so fun that I just have to do it.

We go to a Mexican place we've never been to and I get a margarita. It's good and strong. The food is the best Mexican I've had in town. The boy offers me one of his last chicken nuggets. I think that's wonderful. Maybe he does like me. Maybe I really have been wrong about the whole thing.

Nobody has called us back about the kittens, so we go to the pound. It closes in ten minutes, and we dash through the dog room so the boy can look at the dogs, then check out the cat room. All the kitties are adorable, but the first one I see I fall in love with. She's a gray and tan tortie, six months old, loves me back right away. I want her, but we meet all the kittens just to make sure. I take the tortie out of her cage once more and she purrs and begs me to take her home. I'm happy to comply.

I go to pay $70 on a credit card I shouldn't even have. I have a bad history with credit cards, and had to declare bankruptcy a few years ago with $45,000 in debt. Whenever I tell someone about it, I always add that some of it was medical, but most of it was overspending on credit cards when I was manic, or trying to make myself feel better when I was depressed, or paying bills when I lost jobs because I got sick. I've had over 20 jobs.

I don't know if I'm manic today. I just feel good, really good. And I woke up feeling so bad. I was sure the boy hated me, but now he's crouched by the kitten's cage grinning at me hopefully. I put the last $25 for the adoption on my debit card.

We go straight home from the pound and introduce our new kitty to the bedroom. The meeting with the other kitties will come later. I'm thrilled to have a new cat. I've always felt closer to cats than I have to people. When I'm manic, I think I can communicate with them through thoughts, like telepathy.

When we bring the new kitty to the living room, the other cats are interested. But the new, unnamed kitty growls ferociously back at them. Lots of hissing and growling all through the room ensues, and the kitten dashes to hide under the bed. It makes me nervous. Have I done the wrong thing? Did I go over my credit limit? Is this going to work out? I'm feeling really stressed. I want a beer, but I don't need to be drinking this early, especially with the boy here. I'll wait until we grill later. I think about taking my Xanax, but I don't want to be sedated. I feel too alive today.

Some time passes. I read a little. This book is wonderful, but I'm feeling bad. Did I do something wrong? *Something* feels so wrong, but I don't show it. This is a good day. The boy seems to like me today, the man I love is happy, there's a new kitty.

I get a fish on a string, a cat toy, and coax the kitten out from under the bed, thinking I need to make an effort to make her feel comfortable. The boy comes in and snatches the toy away from me. The kitty wants the toy, but is shy at first. Eventually, her playfulness wins out and the boy and I spend the next hour playing with her on the bed. It makes me feel better but I don't want to change anything so I mostly just sit and giggle.

We grill. I drink a beer. It's drizzling now. The burgers smell great. I love being outside. Everything is okay now. We tell the boy to play with his Star Wars toys in the mud. He's mortified. What if they get dirty? I tell him he can take them in the shower with him. He hunches on a cobblestone and delicately tips a storm trooper's feet into the mud. The boyfriend tells him to take his shoes and socks off and walk in the mud, to get on in there, but the boy is horrified and disgusted with this and doesn't do it.

We eat. I eat fast. I've finished my burger before my boyfriend has even taken a bite. I worry about my weight. I've lost so much since changing from Zyprexa to another medicine. I don't want to gain it back.

> "I don't know if I'm manic today. I just feel good, really good."

The boy plays on the cobblestone with his action figures. I ask him what he's doing and he says he's waiting for someone to come and play with him. It just about breaks my heart, and I want to do something, but what? I tell the boyfriend, and when he's done eating we take off our shoes and sit right in the mud with the boy. I'm smiling as the mud sinks into my pants. I think about being a girl and loving sticking my hands and feet in the mud. I was such a happy child before I got sick.

The boy looks grossed out but curious. He wants to play this way but doesn't know how. It's our job to show him. We start by drowning the Star Wars figures in mud, and then we're slinging mud at each other. There's mud everywhere, and each time we throw some at the boy, he runs into the road looking worried, but highly entertained.

I'm laughing so hard I'm coughing. This is fun! We are weird, maybe, but nobody's driving by and the neighbors can't see us. I wish I could always feel this free. And I just can't stop laughing.

We're out here for an hour or so just playing, and it takes about an hour to clean ourselves and the floors and everything else up.

Now we're going to play charades and we teach the boy how. We decide that we'll make up our own words and the other two will try to guess. When the boyfriend is standing there thinking, the boy says something very inappropriate, and the boyfriend's feelings are hurt. I can't stop laughing and feel like a jerk, but I can't. I'm a jackal, cackling with the hysteria of a lunatic. It's not something to laugh over, but this whole day is too much.

We play a game of memory and I hate it. My memory is terrible. I don't know if it's from the meds or the illness. I used to make straight A's in school, but now I can't remember my last thought.

We put the boy to bed and watch the last two episodes of *Freaks and Geeks*. I'm feeling numb but happy overall. I ponder how I'm always assessing my mood. Am I happy? Too happy? Happy enough? Am I depressed? What do I do about it if it's not just right? Do I sleep? Eat? Take pills? Have a beer? Pet a cat? Something always needs to be done, it seems.

We go to bed and I read until I fall asleep. I wake up later with the new kitten curled up to me, but in a few minutes she tries to get on the boyfriend. He doesn't like it and goes to sleep on the couch for the second night in a row. I hate that, but I don't want the kitten to sleep by herself on her first night with us. It's 3 A.M. and I've been lying here for hours petting her and I realize I don't remember taking my meds. I never forget to take my meds. They are my food, water and sunshine. But I can't take them twice. That's poison. I'm almost positive I didn't, but I'm not going to risk double-dosing. If I didn't take them and miss a day, I'll be off-balance for a few days. I know this.

I slip an Ambien and try to fall asleep and not worry about it, slowly stroking my new kitty's head, hoping that she'll calm down and feel at home eventually. That what I have to give is enough. That maybe someday things will be normal. I have my nightly fantasy about the day a cure comes and I no longer have to swing all over the place. I drift off to sleep to the sound of a happy purr.

Lisa Rusczyk is the author of the novel *The Blue Pen*, published by Club Lighthouse Publishing in 2009. She was diagnosed with bipolar disorder when she was 21.

Psychosis

Stephen Koller

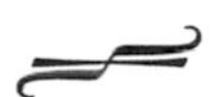

Had a meltdown today. I've been low for some time now. Forgetting to take my meds in the morning and an inappropriate outburst from Caren were all it took to break this mother wide open.

My day began in the ordinary way. Woke up sad. Cursed my horrid C-Pap and went to work. I had a meeting with the guys at Fox Subacute, which was depressing. Guys with Duchenne Muscular Dystrophy who are my own age are an anomaly. None of them have more than a year left, maybe two at best. I can't, for the life of me, figure out what keeps a guy in that predicament going from day to day. I mean, we can all imagine what we would feel if we found out we had only a little time left, but to live your whole life knowing that the chances of making it to your 30s is dim has got to play with your mind in unknowable ways. How can they all have such wonderful senses of humor?

Nevertheless, my rut was wedged ever deeper as I burst from this strange collision of life's journeys back into the sun-scorched outside world. I sat in my car to roll a cigarette when Caren called, screaming some nonsense into my ear that was not meant for me. It was meant for my mother. After a mutually ridiculous verbal skirmish, my mother called with angry nonsense not meant for me; it was meant for Caren. I, once again, challenged the decibel capability of my vocal chords like an obscene, hideous, overgrown child. This time there was no skirmish, no back and forth. There was only the quick death of a conversation. Silence. She had hung up the phone. Once again, as I've done all my life since birth, I had hurt the woman who brought me into this terrible, beautiful world. I was ashamed, even though I knew both she and Caren were in the wrong.

That was it. I tried to call them both over and over to rectify the situation, to converse properly, like an adult. Each time I called, the phone rang like a town crier in a ghost town. Every ring jammed the dagger deeper into my heart.

I did what anyone would do. I entered a state of mild psychosis. Vision inhaled itself into a pinhole. Within mere minutes, the world became an ambient silhouette and my inner voice switched from first to third person.

Driving about 30 miles an hour on the turnpike, my thoughts commanded, *"Kill yourself. Kill yourself. Nobody will help you. Even God has written you off!"*

Time froze as the planet sped in its rotation. I don't remember anything about the 45 minute drive, but I eventually found myself in a Wawa parking lot crying like a baby. I stared at my pocket knife and imagined myself shoving it into my gut and ripping my abdomen open for one final look inside. I saw my stomach walls torn and jagged, revealing a pile of half digested vomit. Intestines slumped out with a wet thud. And finally, all of the sickness would come out of me. All of my failures, embarrassments, secret shames would drop from my corpse to find a new host body to parasitically invade. Once and for all, the noise of my thoughts would cease.

> "Nobody will help you. Even God has written you off!"

Caren called again. She yelled at my mom through my ears again. I blurted some quieter insanity and hung up the phone...again.

"Kill yourself. Kill yourself. Nobody can help you. You're too fucked up."

The thoughts pulsed in verbal melody like the chant of the sick little children in Lord of the Flies. *"Kill the pig. Cut its throat. Spill its blood."*

The knife looked good, but my children look better. This is why I know my psychosis is only mild; I realized my kids need their father for better or for worse.

Caren called again, but this time I got to witness a miracle for the second time in a few weeks: she apologized with sincerity. It didn't fix me, but it did stop the voice's maniacal command. My thoughts returned to first person. I meandered through the remaining hour and a half at work and returned home, morbidly depressed.

I took my meds and the mood gradually began to lift. I spent the remainder of the evening in my garden, bonding my body with the earth as I squished mud between my toes. Caren, Bella, and I ate our first pick of fresh peaches straight off the tree and, for the moment, I was glad to still be alive.

Stephen Kolter is a writer living in the Philadelphia area. His writing is an attempt to understand his symptoms and to converse with others about the illness.

One Sparkling Facet

Natalie B. Rowe

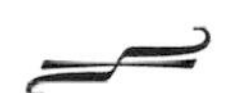

Strange that the staff trusts us with boiling water, I think to myself as I stand in the kitchenette of a hospital psychiatric ward, making myself a cup of tea and peanut butter on toast. My latest medication has turned me into a ravenous foodaholic, resulting in 15 fresh pounds packed onto my normally slender frame. This torments me as much as my unbalanced mental state.

While the tea steeps, I plunk myself down in the fluorescent-lit common area, joining other patients lured in by the mesmerizing boob tube. They look medicated and defeated. Do I look the same? A bathrobe-clad inmate from the "involuntary" ward shuffles past, muttering to herself and looking every bit the stereotypical lunatic. The lighting's greenish cast accentuates her dark under-eye crescents, her sallow skin, her frowsy bed-hair. I hope to God I am looking better than that.

I'm a "voluntary" admission, meaning I signed myself in of my own free will, unlike the wild-haired woman aiming for the kitchen. No straitjackets, chemical restraints or stretchers for me, not even a pillowy padded cell. Patients like me stay in one ward, involuntary admissions (a.k.a. "dragged in kicking and screaming") in another, with different sets of rules and locks. Sometimes we inmates intermingle.

On the advice of my psychiatrist, I'm here for rest, evaluation and an adjustment of my medication. I was having trouble adjusting to the latest in a series of pharmaceuticals that did more to hinder than to help. I spent weeks riding a high punctuated by bouts of agitation, irritation, and recurring thoughts of suicide, an act I contemplated as early as age 10 but have thus far succeeded in resisting. Fireworks of thoughts were exploding in my brain. Nothing stopped the hamster wheel in my head. My worried husband at last took me to my psychiatrist, whom we affectionately (but not to her face) call the "nut-doctor." She spoke gently, sensing my suffering.

"I've never seen you in such a bad state. What would you think about checking into hospital for a rest?"

No objections from me; a respite from my overheated brain sounded divine. Comforting visions filled my head: Florence Nightingale nurses, pastel rooms, cards and bouquets cramming my night table, Caribbean views and fresh ocean breezes.

No ocean breezes in this place, I think as I listen to Mrs. Shufflefoot engage in an animated soliloquy in the kitchenette. Still, feelings of gratitude swell within. However bad things may be, I can still (and want to!) shower, comb my hair and get dressed. No voices in my head are warning me that the toaster is an alien. (*"Bad toaster, bad! I am not going to the mothership with you!"*) My feet clear the ground when I walk, my hands shake only slightly, and not a hint of drool leaks from the corner of my mouth.

Still, I ain't exactly the poster girl for normalcy. And the psych ward isn't the peaceful oasis I had envisioned. At night, I awake hourly when a figure in scrubs (orderly? nurse? pervert in disguise?) unsubtly whips back the curtain and aims a flashlight at me, presumably to ensure I haven't opened up the veins on my wrists, or gargled with Drano.

My dear husband does indeed bring me flowers, and as always holds me close both physically and emotionally, but I'm not keen on entertaining any other visitors. I want as few as possible to know about my sojourn at the "Hotel Crazy-fornia." Thus, the card and posy collection remains small. I try and fail to read a novel. My level of concentration does at least support staring out the window.

Back in the kitchen, the unhinged visitor has procured her snack and pads back to her ward, still wrestling vocally with her brain-demons. She has seen fit to leave the extraterrestrial toaster unscathed, but when I walk up to the counter, I realize my tea has disappeared altogether. The reason is soon clear: Mrs. Shuffle-foot has absconded with my beverage, contained in a mug I'd brought from home! There is nothing to do but turn the kettle back on. I am not about to confront someone who confuses a small appliance with ET.

How has it come to this, that I'm lodged in a psych ward, my beverage stolen by a be-slippered stranger? The road has been interminable and potholed. While most people were greeting the new millennium with champagne kisses and fears of a computer virus that would bring down modern society, I was pondering my shiny new diagnosis: type II bipolar disorder. The "II" means that instead of becoming manic, I reach only hypomania, a lesser sort of high. I've never had psychotic episodes nor been hospitalized involuntarily for my illness. I have, however, experienced uncontrollable mood swings, sometimes exhausting my complete emotional palette in the space of a day. Suicidal thoughts have permeated my brain without invitation, most often when I am depressed but sometimes when I am zippy. While type II is often characterized as a less severe version of the illness, I find that debatable. After all, if you end up dead by your own hand, as many people with this kind do, is it less serious than ending up dead by your own hand, as many people with the "more severe" kind do? Dead is dead.

Diagnosis at age 35 did bring relief: my chaotic brain chemistry finally had a name. It can be hard to ferret out this version of the illness; it's easy to see depression, but hypomania can be mistaken for something more benign, like chattiness, excess charm, or industriousness. While being treated for depression five years earlier, I'd told a psychiatrist about my uncle's bipolar disorder, and that I often felt like a "mini-manic depressive." This comment failed to register, and I continued on with my therapy, waiting for my sadness to lift.

"I felt blighted by my diagnosis and told few people about it."

Besides, I knew I wasn't exactly like my uncle. For starters, I didn't stay up all night for days on end, cleaning my home in a way that would shame Martha Stewart more than her stay in the slammer. My moods didn't soar stratospherically like my uncle's. And unlike some afflicted with this disorder, I luckily never indulged in recreational drugs, drank like a fish or succumbed to promiscuity. I was always responsible with money. And yet there were things about my uncle that reminded me of, well, *me*, and I don't mean our needing glasses.

I recall my father, now gone, speaking of my uncle's treatment disparagingly, telling me that this psychiatric stuff was nonsense, that if his brother would only try harder, be stronger, and pull up his socks, he wouldn't need these zombifying medications. While I didn't think Dad was being fair, part of me took the message to heart anyway. Now I found myself wondering if my own attempts to rein in my galloping emotions had been half-assed. I'd had lots of therapy in my life; why hadn't that been enough to prevent this mental disintegration? Why did my socks keep falling down?

Back on the ward, I mention my missing tea mug to the reception nurse, and she kindly retrieves it. A few days later, my husband takes me home.

While I feel somewhat better, there's a long way to go towards recovery and understanding. I've since found a psychiatrist gifted in pharmaceutical chemistry. He prescribed a drug combination that stabilizes me without hellacious side effects. My sensitivity to psych medications borders on the ridiculous, so it's taken a gentle touch and much tinkering to achieve the right balance. While I still struggle with constant fatigue and a slightly fuzzed brain, the trade off is worth it.

During the nine years since my diagnosis, I have come to a slow, grudging acceptance of my mental illness. While I lead a healthy lifestyle and follow my psychiatrist's advice, I know that a certain part of my bipolar disorder remains beyond my control. Stress is the enemy, so I live a quiet rural life, surrounded by rolling farmland with views that feed the soul. My workspace is at home, where I can create art in my pajamas should I so choose. My great joy is my husband, who has loved and supported me unconditionally throughout this journey.

For a long time, I felt blighted by my diagnosis and told few people about it. Even now the fear of stigma makes me question sharing this side of myself; I can't stand to be judged on a psychiatric label alone. I continue to struggle with extending myself the same sympathy I have for others with this illness. Still, I believe my mercurial brain chemistry is the fuel for much of my creative fire, the force that has shaped me as an artist. It's a stretch to call bipolar disorder a blessing, but without it I think I would feel less, create less and live a lesser life. Bipolar disorder is just one sparkling facet of me, not my definition. I can live with that, and I hope to do so for a very long time.

After graduating from the University of Toronto with a Bachelor of Music degree, Natalie B. Rowe realized that she wasn't cut out to be a classical clarinetist. She now works as a graphic designer, illustrator and fiber artist. Writing remains her first and most passionate love. She met her husband, Gordon Campbell, in the Royal Canadian Naval Reserve, which they joined because it offered travel, food and paying gigs for musicians. Now peaceniks, they live on an 86-acre farm with two dogs, three cats and a gecko. Natalie has illustrated a children's book about a rattlesnake entitled *Katie of the Sonoran Desert*.

So, You Crazy?

Nicole Kafka

Holding my three new prescription slips, I burst off the elevator, pushing past a little old man. Focusing my attention on our car in the parking lot, I sprint forward, leaving my mom to fight the crowd on her own. I flip the car door handle, hoping that the car, like magic, will instantly take me home to my room. Mom reaches the car. I flip the handle harder. Mom unlocks the doors and I slide into the seat, clenching my new prescriptions. These slips of paper make me rethink my decision to finally see this new doctor.

I curl up in the seat as we pull out of the spot and head home to the sanctity of my room. We stop multiple times to let tired parents of small children that not even Super Nanny could help, and many sad-looking men and women, due for their "happy pills," cross the parking lot. I'm drawn to the delusional rants of a young woman, and the horns that are blowing as she pounds on cars in the street. Screaming loudly about the aliens landing at Towson Town Mall and something about Jesus working for the CIA, she dances wildly. As she swings her arms around, laughing, she's no longer a stranger. Her blonde hair and bright smile are transformed into mine, and it's me in the street screaming my delusions. Mom asks me, "What drugs is she on?" and it brings me back to the car. Still clenching my new prescriptions, I mumble,

"Apparently some good ones!" to conceal my terror that someday that person will, in fact, be me.

The light turns green and Mom hits the gas. She reaches over and turns up the radio. Captain and Tennille blares out of the car speakers as Mom sings and moves to the beat of *Love Will Keep Us Together*, while I try not to hear the music.

> *I slouched in my chair and half-heartedly flipped through the Bikers Weekly that was lying on the reception room table, avoiding eye contact with everyone, including my mother. My attention was broken away from the article on Harleys vs. Japanese Made Bikes by an older man calling my name. Seated in his office, we discussed a life of extreme highs and bottomless lows. I listened to my mom tell story after story about my life. Then it was my turn to tell the real version. Febreezing my college roommate at three in the morning; having to leave the mall because there were too many people; calling a friend at 5 A.M. just to say hi; acting out my Mexico trip to the entire cafeteria. The room fell silent except for an occasional sniff from Mom. The older man placed his pen on his desk and leaned back in his chair.*
>
> *"You've told me about your ups and downs; can you tell me about your normal state?*
>
> *I looked at him, puzzled, thinking that he must be joking or that he apparently hadn't been listening for the last half hour. I laughed and shrugged, "That's what I thought I just did." This was my normal, and I had just begun to question it myself.*

"You like my car dancing?" Mom looks over, smiling. I just shake my head. I can't seem to talk right now; everything's spinning out of control. The car slows to a stop in traffic at Northern Parkway, and I watch the young black boy selling ice cold water running in between the cars. I recall passing this street before, months ago as my friend and I drove home at 10 M.P.H., Bonnie's nose inches away from the steering wheel, trying to find the road, as we laughed so hard that tears streamed down our faces. We had left our friends' house knowing neither one of us should be driving because we had downed our usual "party aids" of muscle relaxers and pain killers. As we inched our way down the road, so as to not draw attention from the cops, Bonnie's eyes caught the White Avenue street sign. Smiling to myself, I remember her remarks about the racist street and how there is no Black Avenue, and realize now how ridiculous and out of control our actions really were. Mom, assuming my grins are in light of her car dancing, continues to bounce as the light turns green.

"I am an entity alone in myself, watching other lives being lived."

As we merge onto the Beltway, I feel the car's V6 kick in. In an instant, the speed of the world around me is no longer the same as the speed of the world inside my mind. The trees and other cars zoom by, flashes of color, counterpoints to the slowness of my movements. I am an entity alone in myself, watching other lives being lived, powerless to move into the fast-paced reality. I almost chuckle at the absurdity of opening the car door and letting myself into that world as Mom does 60 M.P.H.

Staring at the door, I contemplated whether microwaving a Hot Pocket to soothe the growling of my stomach would be worth having to move off the bed I had been in for three days. Knowing that even to open the door and make my way the five steps to the bathroom took hours of internal encouragement, I wasn't quite sure if the pain in my stomach was enough to lure me out of my confinement. I fought my way through tear and snot-soaked tissues to sit up, my eyes red and swollen, my hair greasy. I mumbled a few words about what a mess I looked to my dog, the only creature I allowed in my room, and made my way to the door. I placed my ear tightly against the door, making sure I would go undetected; I opened it slightly and peaked out to ensure that the world beyond had been halted, waiting for my entrance.

Taking the off ramp, Mom and I fall into place in the line of traffic. I stare through the windshield and Mom sniffs loudly, announcing, "That guy next to us smells good."

I turned toward him and breathed deeply. The smell of his Adidas cologne filled my head and it hurt. I trusted him; he seemed so nice online, and from what he'd told me in the past fifteen minutes, his muscled, 6 foot 3 inch frame was used for nothing more than helping old ladies cross the street. I told him about my life, starting with pre-K and scraping my knee when Ryan pushed me off the jungle gym, to my dislike of orange Skittles, to where each pair of my shoes "lost its virginity," ending finally with what outfit I wore them.

"You're so nice; I think we should be best friends, Eddie." He laughed and I insisted on skipping our way to the play ground. A bee hovered over my head. I almost expected myself to scream and run, squealing, waving my hands over my head as girly as I possibly could. Instead I found myself grabbing at the bee, dancing around in the wet grass, my flip flops slipping with each turn. I asked my new friend, the bee, if he wanted to join me in my makeshift waltz. Eddie sat down on the concrete step leading to the elementary school, and began to tell me stories of his days as a football star. I tried to listen but I couldn't pull my attention from the leaves that danced in the light summer wind, until I was brought back to reality, the

reality of that night, by the slap of his hand on his knee, exclaiming that "it's scary how something like a knee injury can change a whole life." I shifted my weight around on the concrete step underneath me. The slap turned my mind to an old country song and I started to sing my own words about "your career is over and you're gonna be a bum 'cause you ain't got nothing else." Laughing, I could see my song wasn't as amusing to him as it was to me. Instead of an apology that would normally follow a blunder like that, I pulled myself off the step by the railing onto my feet. My feet slipped as the wet grass invaded my flip flops and I tripped.

"It's past my bedtime; I must be off, please escort me home before I fall down asleep right here." Before I could do my wonderful impression of a dramatic faint, hand on forehead and all, I was being pulled by my wrist toward the woods, through the dirt of the baseball fields. The early morning dew that lay on the grass soaked slowly into my jeans as I tried to wrap my toes around my left flip flop, trying to hold onto it. The snap of the tendons in my wrist pulled me back from my month-long high.

I fought, digging my feet into the soft wet dirt. He chuckled, "If you didn't want this, you shouldn't have come out this late with me." My "natural" high lifted even more, and I could see my body being pulled closer to his spot, that's what he called it. I ran the night's events through my now conscious and sane mind, trying to find my way out.

I walked into the kitchen, one flip flop, wet jeans, and swollen wrist. I grabbed a pink Post-it note and wrote, "I think I do need to see that doctor." I placed it on the cabinet and lay in bed waiting for Mom to wake up and make that call.

I smile and nod as we drive past the guy whose scent had gotten my mother's attention. "Yeah, Mom he does smell good." The surge of wind that blows through the window rustles the forgotten, crumbled prescriptions in my hand. I see my face in the windshield. I know these pills will change my world, but I don't think I'm scared.

Rounding Kittendale Circle, I can hear the classic rock and obscene mumbles of a Saturday of Dad working on the truck. As we pull in, Dad walks over, wiping the grease off of his hands. "So, you crazy?"

Air hugging to avoid the grease, I answer, "Yeah, but what's new?" Knowing that he wants more information, I repeat what the doctor told me this morning. For the first time, I say it aloud:

"I'm bipolar."

Nicole Kafka is psychology major at the College of Notre Dame of Maryland who enjoys writing creative non-fiction.

Ups and Downs

Gareth Allen

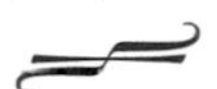

When I was nineteen, I went into the bathroom of my parents' house, locked the door, and removed the lid from the toilet tank. Finding the half-bottle of vodka that I had hidden there that morning, I took a long pull from it. I closed my eyes as I felt the warmth reach across my chest. Sitting down on the toilet, I pulled out my wallet and, with delicate fingers, removed the razor blade from behind my bank card, curious for a moment at my anxiety to avoid cutting my fingers.

When my depression consumed me like this, my usual decision-making functions were buried beneath an impenetrable fog of doubt, despair and unrelenting mental exhaustion. I didn't want to die; that would have been a positive step towards something else. No, I just couldn't be bothered to remain alive. So I sat for a couple of seconds with the blade pressed against the soft, fleshy part of my wrist, just to the side of the knot of tendons. Taking a deep breath, as though I was about to leap off a diving board, I plunged the metal into my skin and made a couple of rough cuts, before deftly swapping hands and repeating the process, the blood already spreading across my lap.

To this day, I don't really know whether it was a genuine suicide attempt, or what is commonly referred to as "a cry for help." It seems that I was so paralyzed by self-doubt, I couldn't even make a commitment to death. How tragic that one's first feeling on being rescued from dying should be disappointment.

I am a salesman. Now 32, I have been selling professionally for half of my life. Since going out into the world and getting a real job, I have turned my hand to selling a variety of products and services: mobile phones, conservatories, sporting equipment, advertising space, insurance. The point is that I am good at it. Very good at it. I realize that this sounds arrogant, and frankly, that's what it is. Because having the confidence to knock on doors–either figuratively or literally–and convince people to give you their money requires a certain arrogance. Giving up money is simply not something that comes naturally to most people.

If I feel proud of my confidence when I am feeling so good, should I not then feel ashamed of my depression when I am stricken by that? Perhaps when I was sitting in that bathroom, I was ashamed. But with the intervening life experience, I have come to realize that these experiences, both positive and negative, are merely part of what makes me the person I am. What I do with those raw materials is what constitutes my achievements.

"I feel vibrant and alive. But I am constantly aware that this is a phase, and that a change will occur."

Since getting my bipolar under control, I still have periods of manic energy, where work and home life occupy my mind non-stop, and I struggle to sleep with the opportunities and ideas whirling around my head. During these periods, I am productive at work, I exercise and lose weight, I feel vibrant and alive. But I am constantly aware that this is a phase, and that a change will occur. The years of experience allow me to manage those changes. With those years of experience to draw on, I can now spot the early warning signs of depression: a sudden lack of energy and enthusiasm, a gnawing, unspecific anxiety deep in my gut, a general sense of dissatisfaction with a life that was rewarding only days earlier.

For example, earlier this week, I attended a small sales seminar which involved an hour of hand-shaking and meeting new people, followed by my giving a ten-minute presentation. If you asked the twenty or thirty people who I met that day to give their impressions of me, I am sure you would find that I got on better with some than with others. However, I would imagine that most of them would have left with an impression of a confident and dynamic young man in full control of his business. I am absolutely sure that none of them would have known the truth: that I spent the previous night tossing and turning in paroxysms of anxiety, that I was so full of self-loathing and distaste that I couldn't bring myself to look in the mirror when I brushed my teeth that morning, and that I had gone through the whole exercise as though having an out-of-body experience.

Having the knowledge to see these things early allows me to manage the symptoms and take the appropriate medical advice. At nineteen years of age, without that experience, I allowed myself to be sucked into a downward spiral that led me to that bathroom with that razor blade.

I've never made a secret of the fact I suffer from bipolar disorder. It's not the sort of thing you casually bring up during a job interview or a first date, but I have always been open about the condition, and particularly how it has affected my life. Because of my condition I can relate to people who campaign for the rights of minorities. It is a virtually invisible disease, and the stigma is such that those without direct experience all too easily dismiss it as "all in your head."

The truth is that bipolar disorder is not "unhappiness," "moodiness," or "the blues." It is a chemical imbalance of the brain which involves the under-production of serotonin. Physically speaking, I suppose this is "all in your head." But, then, so is a brain tumor.

Like all people, I have had occasion to feel deep unhappiness: at the ending of a relationship, the death of a close relative. These feelings are very real and would be very painful to anyone. But to compare these feelings with depression is simply not appropriate. Comparing unhappiness to clinical depression is akin to comparing a stubbed toe with a broken ankle. Not only is depression different from unhappiness, it is not even measured along the same scale.

Two years ago, my wife Pam had our first child. Fatherhood changes every man in ways for which they are not ready, no matter how much they might prepare. Our inherent selfishness is subjugated to the will of this new life form. It's programmed into our DNA–our very reason for existence is the survival and success of our offspring. As soon as Thomas was born, some primordial genetic program was launched which threw everything upside down.

Now, with all my hopes and fears tied up in this extraordinary little man, my greatest worry is that he will inherit this bipolar disorder from me. It is an inheritable disease, so I wrestle daily with the guilt that I may pass on this condition. However, if this comes to pass, I know that it is my role as a father to help him through it. Having this responsibility gives me a renewed sense of purpose, which selling insurance simply can't touch.

I am not proposing that parenthood is the cure for bipolar disorder; in the last two years, I have had peaks and troughs of emotion just as I did before. But now there is a meaning to everything, a reason to keep going through the difficult times, and a sustaining force that I can cling to in the darkest of days.

As I remember that day thirteen years ago when I just couldn't be bothered to go on living, I feel so sad for the sick and confused young man I was. I want to grab hold of him and tell him that there are so many reasons to go on. I want to tell him to fight through the darkness and hang on with all his might, because this experience will make him stronger, and will give him a renewed sense of purpose.

I want to tell him that there is another young man, not yet born, who is going to need him in thirty years' time. Another young man who will look to him for guidance and inspiration. I want to tell him that even now, in this pit of despair, he is already an inspiration. That I could not be what I am today without him.

Gareth Allen has suffered from bipolar disorder since the age of seventeen. In addition to being a successful businessman in the North of England, he works for several mental illness charities. He has been writing for as long as he can remember and finds the catharsis of writing an escape from the daily grind.

There's Always Something More Than Meets the Eye

Sarah Colman-Hayes

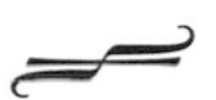

I was in 8th grade when I was diagnosed with Bipolar Disorder II. At the time I was going through a little identity crisis. It's frustrating and annoying not knowing who you are. So I started hanging out with a different crowd. Everything about them was different from that of my previous group of friends. They dressed and acted differently. Their taste in music was different. Even the way they treated people and how they presented themselves was different. I figured *Hey, I'll give it a shot.*

That was a big mistake. Before long, I was dressing and acting just like them. Then I began to think like them. A couple of them talked about cutting themselves. The way they talked about it made it seem like it was no big deal. But the scars that were left after they did it were scary. Some were short and just on the wrist. One of the girls, however, had both her arms covered in long gashes.

One day, my best friend and I had made plans to play against each other in a soccer game. But I had also RSVP'd to attend a Bat-Mitzvah on that same day. My mom and dad told me I had to go to the Bat-Mitzvah because I had already RSVP'd and because it was also more important than a soccer game. I got very upset. Very, very upset. I don't know why, but the image of the scars on that girl's arm flashed in my mind. One minute I was sitting on my bed with angry tears in my eyes; the next my brother was shouting "No! No! No! Don't do it!"

I had gone in to the kitchen, taken my bracelet off my right wrist, pulled out a sharp knife and was just about to press the blade into my wrist. When I heard my brother's voice, I immediately dropped the knife and ran back to my room and closed my door. My dad came after me.

"You need help."

We got help. In the beginning, I thought of myself as a freak. I was embarrassed. I was on medication all day, all the time. "Normal" people didn't have to be medicated, I thought. They could stay up late on school nights and still make it to school on time the next day, and stay up even later during the weekends if they wanted to. I couldn't do any of that. My week days were done by about 6 or 7 P.M. By 8 P.M. I was in bed asleep, 10 or 10:30 on weekends. People took it the wrong way when I said I couldn't hang out, go to the movies, come to their party, etc. I didn't explain why, because I was embarrassed. If I thought of myself as a freak, wouldn't they think that too?

> "The friends I've kept have helped me through some tough times. I hope that someday I can be there for them just like they have been there for me."

I took a year off from school, had to deal with some difficult family issues and had a bad couple of weeks during that year. But I was also able to figure out what kind of career I wanted and how I was going to make it happen.

I'm currently enrolled in cosmetology school and loving every minute of it.

I've been in therapy for more than four years now. I have a psychiatrist whom I see every few months. I'm also on medication. I take antidepressants, anti-anxiety meds and mood stabilizers. My social life has taken a different turn. I lost friends and fell out of touch with a few people. But the people I've stayed in touch with and the friends I've kept have helped me through some tough times. I hope that someday I can be there for them just like they have been there for me.

One thing I have learned on this journey is that even though it may feel to those of us with bipolar disorder like we are alone, we are not. There are many of us, and we all go through a lot of the same emotions and challenges. When I'm having a bad day or week, I remind myself about one thing: If I weren't bipolar, I wouldn't be me!

Sarah Colman-Hayes is 20 years young and lives with her mom and younger brother in sunny Southern California. This is the first time she has written publicly about being bipolar.

PART TWO

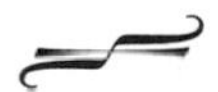

"...they took me out of school, as I could no longer function..."

"...I woke up in a psychiatric hospital..."

"...at last we had a *diagnosis*."

The Girl Who Used To Be Me

Gail Livesay

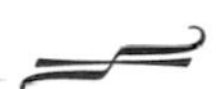

"Come birthday girl, pancakes await."

My cheerful mother tugged at the covers, but I just pulled them up higher over my head. I'd gone to bed the previous night the way any kid would on the eve of her 13th birthday: eagerly anticipating the morning. But I awoke feeling so tired that I wanted to never get up. Later on that day, my mother made a nice dinner with cake and ice cream. But I didn't enjoy my birthday; though no one knew it, I spent much of the day hiding and crying.

I grew up in the sixties, a member of a large farm family, nine in all. We all worked hard and each of us children had chores to do. But money was scarce and we were taken to see the doctor only in the case of a life-or-death emergency or a broken bone.

I had awful bouts of feeling tired and sad. Sometimes I was unable to sleep for days at a time. My parents didn't notice; they worked so hard that they fell asleep as soon as their heads hit the pillow, and they were unaware of what was happening with me at night. They did notice, however, when I started getting into trouble in school. Sometimes I would talk too much, too fast. I'd feel like I could do anything—and sometimes I could. Then there were days I sat through my classes barely aware of what was going on. I felt like three little girls lived inside of me, one tired and sad, one too full of energy, always doing outrageous things, and the one who used to be me.

Things kept getting worse at school. My teachers told my parents I could do my work if I just applied myself, but it wasn't as easy as that, far from it. My mood swings got so bad that Mom and Dad finally took me to see the only doctor in our little farming community, who was quite old. He just attributed my problems to hormones and nerves associated with puberty, and that was the end of that.

> "It was a surprise to everyone when the bright, energetic person I was simply shut down."

Life went on and I tried to cope but I didn't do too well. In high school, I got in with a wild bunch of kids and discovered that drinking eased my pain. I got pregnant at sixteen and had to drop out of school. I was lucky that Wayne, the boy who got me pregnant, wasn't part of my usual crowd. He was kind, a friend of my brother and he married me. We were way too young, but we stuck it out and eventually added another child to the family.

I went through several years where the sadness lessened, and I became driven—driven enough to accomplish a lot. I got my GED and went to business college at night while working at Kentucky Fried Chicken during the day. I would fix supper for Wayne and our children, Lisa and Michael, study a couple of hours, go to school and usually studied some more before going home to bed. Despite all this I managed to graduate, making the dean's list the whole time I was in college.

I had no problem getting a good job. As with everything else I was an overachiever in this as well, and I was promoted to supervisor in a short time. I was riding a high of success, and though taking the position would require my working third shift, I gladly threw myself into the new responsibilities. This would be my downfall—or maybe my salvation.

Wayne and I were doing really well financially and had just bought a new home. Working third shift allowed me plenty of time to work on my new home and spend time with my family in the evenings and catch a couple of hours sleep before work. Of course, my husband thought I was sleeping during the day, but I wasn't. I was "burning the candle on both ends" in my zeal to keep moving forward.

It was a surprise to everyone when the bright, energetic person they knew me to be simply shut down one day. It was a Saturday. I dropped the kids off at their friend's house to play and drove to meet a friend at her home for a swim, but at a stop sign on the way there, my mind went blank. Blank. I didn't know which way to go or how to drive the car. I felt an awful tiredness radiating through my body and brain. I simply couldn't function any more. I heard horns blaring and people yelling at me as though from a great distance. I guess someone recognized me and called Wayne. I felt him take me from my car and gently place me into his.

I woke up a psychiatric hospital, where I would have to stay for some time. I was diagnosed with bipolar disorder and was given ECT (electro convulsive therapy) to bring me out of my deep depression. The treatments worked, with no ill effects except taking some of my memory away. The doctor advised that I take disability retirement and I was put on medication.

I'm still on the medication. I have therapy sessions every two weeks. I still have bouts of depression and mania, but I'm able to cope much better. I am learning to recognize the signals so that my medicine can be adjusted if needed. God has given me—or has allowed me to have—bipolar disorder, but I have discovered some gifts He has given me along with it, gifts I might otherwise have ignored. Since I have taken time to pause for a few moments, I have discovered there's an artistic streak inside me. I've discovered the joy of writing. I have written some poetry and a play which have been published. I have learned to play the piano and I have gotten to experience the joys of a once-in-a-lifetime relationship that can weather any storm. Wayne and I may have been "too young" when we married, but two children and forty years later we're still together. Although I "lost" many years of potential happiness waiting for a diagnosis and proper treatment, I feel I've gained so much, too.

I have heard it said, "when one door closes, a new one opens." I believe this is true. I'm living proof.

Gail Livesay lives in Berea, Kentucky with her husband Wayne. They have two children, Lisa and Michael, and have been blessed with two granddaughters, Marina and Hannah. Gail is currently writing a memoir about growing up with bipolar disorder.

A New Painting

Sandy McPheron

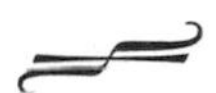

Mental illness is a thief, one that sneaks in and steals the beautiful painting of the life you've imagined for yourself, carefully crafted with just the right images and colors. It stole mine. Before I discovered this thief and banished it, it almost robbed me of that life.

It crept up, cleverly disguised as common depression. Fatigue was the first sign that it had gained entry. Fatigue did not alarm me at first. It seemed logical, given the whirlwind pace of my life at the time. I was a wife, a mother of three, and held a full-time job in addition to working as a school board member. God, what exhaustion! No amount of sleep would relieve it. As it worsened, my appetite faded; everything began to taste like cardboard. Despite the exhaustion, I began to have a hard time sleeping, and spent my nights feeling as if there were dark demons visiting me. If I slept at all, I would wake early, dreading the coming day. I went to my family doctor thinking I might be anemic or showing the first signs of menopause. He drew gallons of blood, but the tests said no.

The thief took his next step—a bold one—when I was on my way home one night. I had what seemed like the most sensible urge to drive my car off an overpass. Even though the urge to do so seemed strangely "normal," I knew something was terribly wrong. I returned to my doctor, who suggested that I was probably suffering from depression. He prescribed some medication which would take four to six weeks to take effect. Four weeks passed, six, then eight as I waited for this magic pill to rescue me, but there was no improvement; in fact, I was feeling worse. My exhaustion was devastating. I ached all over and even moving was difficult. I could not concentrate on the mounds of memos, charts, graphs and budget reports I needed to absorb for work and for the school board. To my exhausted mind they all looked like hieroglyphics. Functioning at home was becoming just as difficult. My husband and kids picked up the slack, taking over the cooking and cleaning, but I wanted to be a wife and mother—the most cherished of the many hats I wore.

> "I felt a faint glimmer of hope as I realized that at last we might have found what was really wrong with me."

A trip to a psychiatrist yielded a different medication but not different results. I was sure everyone was feeling I should just pull myself up by my bootstraps and have a little backbone. I felt this way too, ashamed and angry that I wasn't stronger than this "thing." I tried to hold myself together with the emotional barbed wire and mid-western glue I was brought up with, but it was no use. I felt like I was drowning. Meanwhile, intense anxiety entered my life, binding up my brain and consuming the last of my spirit.

At the recommendation of a friend, I sought the help of a therapist. My hope was that as a team, the psychiatrist and therapist could bring me back to my old self. But I didn't realize that my old self was already gone forever. I didn't know yet that my career, my relationships and my health would be forever changed.

Depression didn't just sap me of my energy and self esteem but also of my judgment, and as a result I stayed with this medical team for five years, by which point they had me on 18 pills a day. My exhaustion and anxiety became mixed with a terrible dash of unpredictable rage, and I completely lost the ability to focus and complete a task. Fearing that I would commit suicide and expose their practice to a lawsuit by my family, the medical team finally referred me to other doctors. So there it was. I was fired as a patient! The parting was very bitter for all, but it would ultimately lead to the correct diagnosis of my condition and my healing under other doctors' care.

The search for a new doctor turned out to be simpler than I thought it would be. I stumbled onto my new psychiatrist with my first interview! He began to ask me questions—questions not just about my bad days, but especially about my good days. I told him about those few wonderful days when I got so much done: laundry, paperwork, projects I had started and not completed, general cleaning and more. Finally he looked at me and said, "Sandy, I think you are bipolar." I was stunned. *Bipolar*? But then I felt a faint glimmer of hope as I realized that at last we might have found what was really wrong with me. He probed me about rage, anger, racing thoughts, anxiety, lack of focus, jumping from project to project, and lack of organization. I answered yes to all of it. All symptoms of what I was to learn was my mania.

He immediately changed my medication, adding lithium, and sent me home with some relaxation tapes to help with my intense anxiety. Over the following months I would come to better understand my manic symptoms. I began keeping mood charts and saw how erratic my moods were. I thought about all the time I had wasted with my former doctors. Why hadn't they questioned their own, obviously flawed diagnosis?

Believe me, there wasn't a sudden "Pow" of wellness. In fact, when this life-saving doctor retired, it took two more psychiatrists and a suicide attempt before I found a new doctor with the right personality—and the right combination of medications—before sanity was achieved. I also had to work to find a compatible therapist and, with effort, I did. I fought hard for my health. And I won.

The other part of my healing came after we moved from our old suburban home of eighteen years into a mountain home called Towering Oaks, named for the three giant oaks in the back yard. Banks of purple periwinkle surrounded the house. Rose bushes dotted the property and weeping birches stood like bookends at the front and back of the house.

There was an orchard of fruit trees in the back yard, and they provided me with the most rewarding therapy. In my more lucid moments, I researched the care of the trees, and I would climb into their branches in the winter to prune them. I found great peace in this activity. Being among my beloved trees, feeling the canyon winds on my face centered me and brought back a long-lost sense of focus. The times in the orchard were wonderful, but sometimes I still had to push myself, preferring to lie on the couch. When I couldn't bring myself to get out there, the picture windows facing my orchard screamed out my failure. But at harvest time the trees yielded their thanks for my more motivated days with an abundance of riches for family, neighbors and friends.

My mental and physical strength grew with each season, and I added vegetable and flower gardens. Slowly, ever so slowly, with the help of my new doctors, a correct diagnosis and my mountain home, I began to heal and find some peace for my troubled mind. I "waited out the demons" and ultimately prevailed.

It was difficult, and at times it still is difficult, not to mourn the years that were stolen from me: that painting of what I once thought life was supposed to be. I haven't replaced the exact painting stolen by that thief, but I've made the space to hang a better one. So I sit on my mountain among my trees, watching the sun rise and fall, the seasons come and go. There I gather a new palette of colors and new images and visions for my new painting.

Sandy McPheron is the mother of three grown children and the grandmother of three. She lives with her husband and dog in the mountains of Southern California.

What They See Is What You Get: On the (Mis)Diagnosis, Un-Diagnosis, and Re-Diagnosis of Bipolar Disorder

J.P. Whetsell

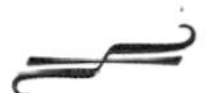

Every teacher I've ever had, every boss, every family member, every friend, virtually every person I meet has his or her own story about me. Every doctor I have ever seen has a story about me as well. But the stories we tell about ourselves are the most important. They affect how we understand our past, how we live our present, and what we believe we can do in the future. But next to my stories about myself, the stories the doctors tell are the most important ones, because they come with diagnoses.

Diagnoses are labels; they are also interpretations that help frame the events of a person's illness. Because my identity is so bound to my experiences with bipolar disorder (seventeen years now, or more than half my life), it is important for me to understand my diagnoses in order to understand myself and the story of my life. The diagnoses can't change the past. But they can shape how I remember events and affect the choices I make. And they can potentially limit my future.

As a writer, having a bipolar diagnosis as part of my identity is even more complex because of the link, both real and romanticized, between mental illnesses and creativity. The list of artists known or thought to have bipolar disorder is long and illustrious, and includes the poet Baudelaire, the composer Beethoven, and the painters Munch and Van Gogh. There are times I wonder how much am I really ill? How much do I want to be ill, or enjoy the idea of being ill, especially if it makes me feel more special or artistic?

Every time I have another episode, I begin questioning myself, my experiences, and my life. There have been times when I was extremely irritable for no good reason and had outbursts of anger. Was that evidence of hypomania? Or merely a bad temper? And if it was a bad temper, was that learned from the adults I had as role models or was it a sign of a borderline personality? I don't think such questions will ever be answered, but I doubt I will ever stop asking them.

People who ultimately wind up with a bipolar diagnosis often go undiagnosed or misdiagnosed for an average of eight to ten years. And, maddeningly, there is a spectrum of bipolar disorders with two currently diagnosable types (I and II), and even within subtypes peoples' experiences are varied. Because my symptoms have been relatively mild and vague at times, or fitting some aspects of multiple disorders, they have been interpreted differently by different people. The school physician deemed me a pathological attention-getter. One therapist thought a diagnosis of personality disorder was appropriate. Depression was quickly recognized by doctors as being my biggest struggle (as is the case for most people with mood disorders), but what type of depression (i.e., bipolar versus unipolar) has been hotly debated by family, friends, and mental health professionals, particularly when I have a new episode or get a new doctor.

At first, my depression and I seemed easy to understand. I cried a lot, spent a lot of time in bed, and ate little. Psychological tests taken one winter rated me high in depression and introversion. The verdict: major depressive disorder. During that spring I made a crisis call, but at my follow-up appointment a few days later I had absolutely no idea what had upset me enough to make that call. Aha! Cyclothymia is the problem, the doctor pronounced. At the beginning of the summer, my new psychiatrist decided I didn't really have any problems that needed pharmacological solutions at all. "It's just adolescence," he declared, "What she really needs is time."

A few years after that, a doctor mentioned to my mother that thyroid problems can cause mental problems like depression in people who are already susceptible. "It was all the Graves' Disease," became my mother's mantra.

During my sophomore year of college, I finished no fall semester classes and started and quickly dropped classes in the spring. I began seeing a new psychiatrist who initially diagnosed me with: *Major Depressive Disorder, Severe, With Psychotic Features*. My doctor and I, although we worked well together for about five years, never discussed this diagnosis; I learned of it by looking up the code from the insurance bills. At first it felt empowering to drive to the library and look up my diagnosis by myself. But later I didn't feel so good about it. What *were* my psychotic features, since they weren't delusions or hallucinations? More than ten years after the fact, it's almost impossible to know what my doctor meant by the diagnosis.

> "I need to be able to tell my story... and to have it believed."

At some point my diagnosis changed to Bipolar Disorder NOS and Dissociative Disorder NOS. My bipolar symptoms were hypomania–the less colorful sister of Bipolar I's hallmark mania–and mixed episodes, which are depressive and manic symptoms simultaneously. My experiences ranged from near-catatonic depressions to nights when I stayed up all night reading or doing needlework. I also spent money much too quickly, mostly on relatively non-extravagant purchases such as compact discs and books. Worse, I lost confidence in my emotions and my ability to express them. When I felt good, I asked myself if I felt *too* good. When I felt sad, I asked myself if I was becoming depressed. Because I was constantly asking myself what and how I felt, I never really felt anything except confusion and worry.

About ten years after my last bout of hypomania, my new doctors said I didn't need a mood stabilizer because I did not have bipolar disorder. Instead, they believed that I had likely been misdiagnosed bipolar in the past because of personality traits that could be worked on through therapy. This was quite a shock to me, as I had lived under a bipolar diagnosis for a decade. Were my family members who insisted I was not bipolar right after all? Was I indeed misdiagnosed bipolar because I really had a personality disorder? Or was it possible I had both? My thyroid had been off balance; did that cause my symptoms? Certainly no psychiatrist ever asked when I last had my thyroid levels checked when I presented with mood symptoms

After I was discharged from the hospital, yet another new psychiatrist said it was impossible for doctors to determine whether someone was bipolar based on a one-week hospitalization for depressive symptoms. Thyroid imbalance could produce anxiety or depression but not the kind of increases in goal-directed behavior I experienced. Her diagnosis, based on my history and careful examination: dissociative disorder and a bipolar illness. The same diagnoses I had in college.

A doctor once asked me how I felt about possibly having bipolar disorder. She said I shouldn't be ashamed, that it was no different from having hypertension or diabetes, and equally controllable. I wasn't ashamed. But if I had hypertension, the illness itself wouldn't change my moods, an integral part of our inner experience. If I were writing about diabetes, I wouldn't consider publishing this essay under a pseudonym. If I had arthritis, I wouldn't make up excuses for going to the doctor so often. If I had some other chronic illness, I wouldn't question every time I deep-cleaned my house or felt like going dancing or was irritable or giggly or felt like staying in bed.

So no, bipolar disorder is not like other chronic illnesses. I now feel pretty comfortable with the diagnosis because it was given by different doctors at different times in my life. In some ways the diagnoses are just labels, but in other ways they tell the story of what's gone wrong and what I need to do to put my life back together. I don't know exactly what combination of genetics, brain chemistry, attitudes, experiences, and beliefs caused my illness or what changes are needed for my recovery. I know, in part, I need to be able to tell my story, if only to myself and to my family. And to have it believed.

Which brings me to a recent conversation with a friend. I told her that my doctors had gone full circle and that I'd been diagnosed bipolar again.

"Oh," she said, "I never doubted you were."

J. P. Whetsell is a graduate student working towards a Masters degree in public health. She lives in North Carolina with her two rabbits.

A Little Help from My Friend

Maria Norman

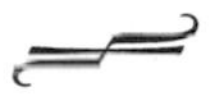

When I was young child my mother used to say, "You're always so nervous." She might have called me something far different had she witnessed a "nervous" episode years later when, my mind driven by bipolar disorder, I viciously attacked my boyfriend to the point of drawing blood.

When I was young, my family teased me for seeming to get mad for little or no reason. As a young adult, a friend once described me as a "shook up can of soda with the lid on." I just thought I was a "Type A" personality. I categorized myself as an extremist. Everything was either all or nothing with me, never any middle ground, especially when it came to partying or spending money.

During the years I was building my tech career, I had highly productive periods that made me the "star," but I was no star in terms of personality. I was intolerant of other people, irritable, and had an insufferable attitude of superiority with delusions of grandeur. At the time, that mood was just "normal" for me.

My personal relationships were disastrous. I always picked the wrong guy. I was seemingly together, with beauty, brains and a killer body, but I invariably picked the losers: no careers to speak of, drug or alcohol addicted. Parasites. I married one of them and was divorced in less than three years, but of course as far as I was concerned it wasn't me who was to blame.

When I was 33, I moved to Silicon Valley from New York City for a big job promotion. I was in another destructive relationship filled with cocaine and alcohol. This person came to live with me, and I slowly spiraled into a period of vicious manic cycling that persisted for over a year. I was miserable, yet successful in business.

The end came when I simply lost it during yet another one of our abusive arguments. He started poking, me which was always the prelude to my getting hit. For the first time something snapped inside me and I threw my first punch. Despite his being 6'4" and 200 lbs of lean, strong muscle, I literally "saw red" and attacked him with my fists, nails and any part of my body that could inflict harm. The neighbors called the police, who hauled both of us away (separately) to the station. I was bloodied, had a fat lip and my stomach and legs were badly bruised. My partner told the cops I hit him first, so I was thrown in jail and a restraining order was issued against me.

Needless to say, the relationship ended that night, but the event continued to haunt me. I began to realize there might be something wrong with me, but denial can be a very addictive drug when it's used as a way of coping with pain.

After that there was a long period of relative stability, more therapy and happy results when I met a great guy who became my husband and, later, father to my two children. All was good until the dot com bust, which tanked his business and forced me to become the primary breadwinner. During that same autumn, 9/11 occurred and I lost many of my childhood firefighter friends. Living so far away from Ground Zero made me feel helpless and unsupportive. Then I lost my best friend to cancer. At that time I was globe trotting as a high level executive while also juggling young children, paying the bills and dealing with a frustrated spouse and the demands of a stressful job.

Things began spiraling down once again—the irritability and mood swings with the children and constant arguments with my husband about every little thing, including his inability to provide for our family. On my forty-fifth birthday I opened a card from his mother that contained what I perceived to be an unnecessary and hurtful comment. When I confronted my husband and started blaming him for his mother's behavior, he responded by saying something extremely rude about my dead mother, whose only crime was to love him and accept him into our family. I saw red again and struck him. The shock on his face is something I will never forget.

> "For the first time something snapped inside me and I threw my first punch."

I immediately went to a psychiatrist, and was diagnosed as Bipolar II. It was a life-altering moment for me. For the first time I realized there was a reason for all those roller coaster moments: the tendency towards violence when triggered, the depression, the weight gain, the poor judgment. I wanted to be—*had* to be—stable to put my life and family back together again and move forward.

Lamictal saved my sanity. Yes, I hate being dependent on medication. Yes, I hate being put in the category of the mentally ill. Yes, I hate the fact that I can't get medical insurance due to a preexisting condition and have to pay almost $400 each month for a 30-day supply of pills.

But I have my family back, can set my priorities more intelligently, and have finally retired from a successful tech career to focus on myself and my health for the first time in my life. Today, I am a highly functional adult with bipolar disorder who can identify triggers and avoid self destructive behavior with a little help from my friend, Lamictal.

Maria Norman was born in Rockaway, New York and lived in and around Manhattan for 31 years. In the early nineties, a professional opportunity brought her to the Silicon Valley to pursue a career in the high technology industry. She is married with two children and runs her own consulting business.

The Struggle and the Hope

Valerie Avrutis

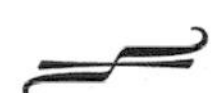

From the time I was a teenager, I knew something was wrong with my moods, which cycled from high to low. A psychiatrist told me that it simply had to do with my being a teenager. In my 30's, I was treated for depression for the first time by my gynecologist. He suggested I see a psychiatrist, who promptly advised me to "grow up and everything would be alright."

In spite of my moods, I thought I could do anything. Succeeding was my only goal and I proved it every day. As a real estate broker I worked endless hours selling land, leasing shopping centers and selling multi-million dollar properties while volunteering in the community. At the same time, I volunteered as project manager of food concessions for a national jazz festival, a perfect match for my energy. The festival required me to fulfill the concession needs of 10,000 people over four days. I planned, scheduled and managed hundreds of hours of volunteer time. As soon as the event was over, the planning began again for the upcoming year. It was a never-ending effort that I eagerly pursued.

When I turned 36, my career changed and so did my mood. My then-husband and I started a custom clothing business. We grew the business from our small home office, working all hours of the day and night. But my as-yet undiagnosed bipolar disorder was affecting every aspect of my life. My husband and I had long, drawn-out fights over big ideas and little problems. My dearest friends were repulsed by my indifference to them and the outrageous language that spewed from my mouth. Where once I was undefeatable, now it was a nightmare being me. Everything seemed like a hassle. Long-term depression set in.

The depression was all consuming and I started spending more and more time in bed. Somehow, I managed to hide the highs and lows from my teenage daughter. The only thing that kept me from killing myself was the thought that she would know I committed suicide. That didn't keep me from praying every night that God would take me. My daughter would be able to accept that, I thought.

It was clear that I needed help, but neither my husband nor I understood the problem or knew what to do. My marriage failed as we drifted farther and farther apart emotionally. He finally told me he wanted a divorce, though it was the last thing I wanted.

Between my depression and losing the love of my life, I couldn't work for over a year. I couldn't get out of bed. I had no self esteem and felt beaten down by life. I was no longer the driven, successful person I once was. The divorce left me alone and without friends. I moved from the $300,000 home my husband and I built together to a rented room in someone else's house.

"I was committed for four days against my will, with no legal rights."

But on the very day I moved out of the house, I had my first stroke of good luck—although I didn't see it that way at the time—when I was diagnosed with bipolar disorder. I considered myself crazy and was unable to absorb what that meant. Lithium was the prescribed drug but I refused to take it because it spelled mental illness to me. Another prescription I had never heard of was given to me. Even with taking this new drug I refused to confront my new reality. My daily up-and-down cycling was obvious to anyone except me, even after I finally agreed to take medication.

Holding a "real" job was out of the question, so I lived off menial service jobs and the remains of the squandered funds from my divorce. I cleaned houses during the day and delivered newspapers at night. I had one episode after another while the concoction of prescriptions was being fine tuned. I hallucinated that my psychiatrist was flying a magic carpet in front of my bed. I imagined a swarm of bees were attacking my genitals. Days on end I would lie in bed sweating, unable to move or eat. I didn't understand how necessary it was to take the drugs regularly. My inconsistency was killing me little by little. During the "good times" I tried to work, smoked cigarettes (though I'd never smoked before) and had wild, crazy sex with strangers.

My doctor kept working to find the right drugs to help me. She and my sisters promised to try to keep me out of the hospital, which was my biggest fear. Finally, the meds started to work and I had a reprieve that lasted a few years. I met and married a wonderful man, Colin, who would watch over me during future horrific episodes. During those episodes, razors were my only thoughts. Colin seemed to know when he could leave me alone and when to stay close. He was and still is my lifeline.

The doctor's nurse practitioner, Deb, took over my care. My episodes became fewer and farther between—until, one night, the worst happened. While my husband slept, I took a handful of tranquilizers and drank vodka, hoping to never wake again. When Colin found me in the morning, I was alive but incoherent. He called my sister, who is also bipolar. She threatened to have me committed to a psych floor if my husband didn't immediately take me in for treatment.

This episode was about to change my life for the better. I was committed for four days against my will, with no legal rights. I was put in a locked-down facility with no way out. I had become one of the truly insane. Trying to commit suicide brought these episodes to a new level and I felt like no one could help me. I spent my time saying prayers, in counseling, and playing dominos. When the doctors asked me questions about my feelings, I gave them the answers I knew they wanted to hear, hoping I could get out sooner.

My daughter, who was now an adult and well aware of my illness, flew to town and braved my fury at still being alive. She took me to see Deb on my release from the hospital. I felt like I had been betrayed by everyone, but especially by Deb. I was crazy furious that she committed me to the hospital. My rage was endless. After crying, screaming—and after many hugs and words of encouragement from her—the fury abated and the healing began.

Deb changed all of my medications to the same medications of my sister. Apparently what works for one family member can work for another. I've had a few glitches here and there, but for the last four years I have been free of those horrific episodes.

Hope has crept into my life. I am happily married to the same man who helped me through that last excruciating episode and I take joy in my relationship with my daughter and new grandson. My career has changed again, but this time I am happy. I've been working for eight years with a family-run fine jewelry store where my efforts are rewarded. My employer and co-workers know of my bipolar disorder and care about me and my well being. These supportive people, along with my medical care, help me accept each and every day.

Valerie Avrutis lives a peaceful, happy life in St. Petersburg, Florida with her husband, Colin. She enjoys writing and spending time with her family.

My Vision of Recovery

Shannon C. Flynn

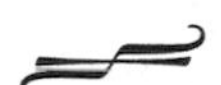

As I entered my senior year of high school, I found myself convinced for no good reason that I was going to die soon, an incontrovertible intuition that I was not long for this world. At that early point I was not contemplating suicide; my sense that God was angry at me and would arrange for a brutal death simply developed into an ever-greater certainty.

Paradoxically, I was at once dreading my death and plunging myself recklessly into life. It seemed to me urgent to design and conduct surveys among my classmates and teachers on handedness and creativity; to cut up and stitch patches on my Catholic girls' high school uniform; to attend 6:00 A.M. mass every morning after staying up most of the night attempting to read ancient Greek history while drinking cold black coffee with salt and pepper sprinkled in it, then before daybreak to wander down the street in my nightgown.

This bizarre behavior and agitation soon subsided, however, only to be replaced by an all-encompassing lethargy that crept into my pores. I found myself less and less able to maintain my demanding schedule of attaining straight A's at my college-preparatory high school, working 25 hours a week at a local store, and generally acting strange.

The proverbial final straw came in the form of the intense pressure and stress brought on by the looming prospect of college applications, for which I was supposed to be preparing by researching and visiting several colleges and universities. While my parents puzzled over my inertness, I simply did nothing to secure a spot at any college whatsoever. I felt incapable of even picking up a university brochure and writing away for a catalog, let alone arranging a visit to a campus, asking a teacher for a recommendation, or crafting an essay. My senior year of high school should have been one of the most exciting times of my life as I readied myself for the four years ahead. Instead, I sank deeper and deeper into a mire of sloth and despair.

My once straight A's became B's, and then C's and D's, and I couldn't even make myself care. I began to detach myself from the world more and more, and to think about death again, this time not as something God was planning for me, but as something that I could plan for myself as the only way out from under the merciless black cloud that hung over me relentlessly. Formerly banal household objects like scissors and vegetable knives took on the sinister promise of ending my melancholy and thick-headed confusion. I took to climbing out on the second floor roof outside my bedroom late at night and talking woefully to myself, all the while wondering exactly how much damage I might do to myself if I jumped. Only my base cowardice kept me from acting on any of these impulses—until I became sicker still and started secretly punching holes in my wrist with pins and paper clips. I didn't cause myself any serious injury, but I told myself I was practicing for the time when the pain became too excruciating and I would finally have no other choice but to act.

One of my most vivid memories of those days is the weekend afternoon my parents lectured me about not having taken a single step toward getting into college, despite the fast-approaching deadlines. "Are you on drugs?!" my dad asked, sincerely baffled. My response was telling: I immediately broke down in a flood of tears, completely ashamed that my own parents could think I would ever take drugs. A normal adolescent response might have been one of indignation or denial, but though innocent of the accusation, I felt only guilt, shame and a deep sense of unworthiness. I must, I thought, be even more evil than I had believed.

"In time, I lifted my head from the floor, spoke to people, and even smiled and laughed again."

This may have been the wake-up call they needed to realize I was in need of serious help. But if my parents didn't read the neon signs then, a few weeks later they had no choice but to accept that I was no longer their golden girl. It was a blustery, rainy November morning. I trudged the few blocks to school as usual, only to experience a sudden but utterly crushing panic after reaching my homeroom. I couldn't breathe, I trembled convulsively, and my heart pounded insistently. I floated outside myself, convinced I would die any moment. My single, consuming need was to *escape*.

As the first class bell rang, I rushed out of the building and, without thinking, half-ran, half-walked down the meandering streets of our neighborhood. I found myself at a bus stop and a city-bound bus appeared. On a whim, I decided that I would ride to the college dormitory of an older friend on whom I had a rather delusional crush. The fact that I didn't have any idea of his address and that he had certainly never invited me to visit him never figured into my chaotically unbalanced equation. I was in a panic for the entire ride, then paced unfamiliar streets in the pounding rain with no umbrella and no more money, until, in need of shelter, I finally stopped at an apartment building. Obviously I was unable to locate my friend, but with psychotic anti-logic I reasoned that if I hung around the apartment vestibule, I could gain enough time to calm down and figure out how to permanently run away from my intolerable life.

My nebulous "plans" were ruined when, after about half an hour, the apartment manager entered the lobby and discovered her disheveled, confused, and frightened squatter. She questioned me repeatedly about my identity, my home address and parents' names and phone numbers, and tried to pry from me why and how I had ended up alone in her building in a rather seedy part of the city. At first I was too paranoid and too incoherent to respond, but I finally broke down and told her the bare facts.

Immediately afterward, the apartment manager called my parents to reassure them I was safe, and then the police, who had apparently been searching for me. I know I was barely connected to reality at the time, but I do remember her comment to the police: "She's obviously emotionally disturbed."

That was an understatement.

My parents arrived and brought me home. They shed tears of relief at finding me, but had no choice but to face my deterioration. I had passed the point of being able to cry and silently fumed that I had not been allowed to escape from the life that was suffocating me. During an emotionally-charged discussion of the incident, I was unable to explain why I had run away from school so suddenly, or indeed to say much of anything to them.

Shortly thereafter, they took me out of school, as I could no longer function there. After a couple of increasingly desperate weeks of round-the-clock monitoring, which was barely sufficient to stop me from acting on my suicidal impulses, my parents brought me to a local psychiatric hospital.

I secretly sighed in relief: for some reason I welcomed the hospitalization. I knew I needed to be in a completely safe place where I could be treated intensively with medications and therapy. But just as important, I wouldn't have to worry about the schoolwork I was missing, the colleges I hadn't applied to, and the family whose love I experienced as intrusive. That I would still be left with my delusions of being evil, my urges to hurt myself, and the overpowering gloom, didn't occur to me.

Twenty-five years later, I can still summon the memory of that awful first night in the hospital. A pleasant but impersonal nurse conducted an interview—to me, an interrogation—about my psychiatric history, probing with particular detail into my suicidal ideation and actions. Upon determining that I was indeed a suicide risk, she plopped a mattress and blanket on the floor of the "quiet room" and told me to get some sleep. The doctor would examine me in the morning. It was the day after Thanksgiving, but I didn't feel I had anything to be thankful for. I hadn't escaped my private hell after all.

As had been customary for the last few months, I barely slept that night, instead ruminating about my fundamental evilness and wincing at the occasional yells of the other patients. Teenagers with all sorts of diagnoses were lumped together in my unit: boys with substance abuse who "acted out" (and who intimidated me beyond reason); pregnant girls whose families had given up on them; and other kids like me with depression, mania and/or florid psychosis all shared this crowded corridor. The first morning after my all-night vigil, I was ordered awake by another nurse and told to take a shower. Immediately I was filled with bewildered anxiety: I hadn't been able to shower or bathe in at least a week and had no inclination to do so now; on the other hand, if I didn't obey these authority figures, who knew what would happen? In the end, I haphazardly unpacked my belongings in the room I'd share with two other girls and slumped on the bed until called to breakfast. Left blessedly alone for a few minutes, I banged my head as forcefully yet as quietly as I could against the bedroom wall. I was not discovered and decided maybe later I'd get a chance to jab my wrist with another safety pin. This, alas, was not to be, as staff members soon examined me, discovered my puncture marks and knew what to watch out for.

For days I wouldn't speak, and when I finally did, I hung my head low and could not make eye contact with anyone, staff or peer. In between encountering frightening teenagers and negotiating group therapy, where I was forced to actually speak and give my name and the reason I was there, I met with my new psychiatrist, a man who looked astonishingly like the college boy I'd tried vainly to visit the day I'd shot out of high school in a panic. *This must be a sign*, I told myself. *The object of my crush has transformed into this doctor who will solve all my problems.* My hopes were dashed over the next few weeks, however, as I came to discover that this "magical" psychiatrist had no patience for my earnest recitation of my psychotic symptoms, dismissing my delusions and ruminations and admonishing me "not to think about that." Still, as the month between Thanksgiving and Christmas progressed, I assimilated into the adolescent ward culture despite myself. I learned to mingle with most of my fellow patients, even some of the loud boys.

I emerged from my bipolar disorder with the help of a drug cocktail of antidepressants, antipsychotics and lithium, and through my participation in art therapy. In time, I lifted my head from the floor, spoke to people, and even smiled and laughed again as my depression and psychosis improved.

My family regained their beloved daughter and sister and I regained my identity, a richer and brighter one filled with hope. This hope has carried me through countless mood episodes and led me to my calling: helping others living with mental illness heal as I have been healed. That's my vision of true recovery.

Shannon C. Flynn obtained a Bachelor of Arts degree in psychology, a Master's degree in art therapy, and a certificate in counseling. She plans to gain licensure as a professional mental health counselor and go on for a Ph.D. in clinical psychology.

PART THREE

"...Mom seems out of control..."

"...I say goodbye to my son as they carry him off on a stretcher..."

"...bipolar is in our blood."

My Mother's Keeper

Patricia F. D'Ascoli

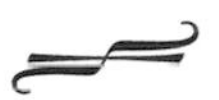

Mom has lost her mind.

At least that's how it seems to me as I pull our Ford Country Squire out of the driveway on a steamy July afternoon. Despite a chilly blast from the air conditioner, sweat slowly trickles down my back; my legs stick to the vinyl seat. Glassy-eyed and silent, Mom sits next to me staring out the window. I wonder what she is thinking, if she is thinking at all.

With knees shaking and heart pounding, I resist the urge to cry. I am 19, but I have somehow been charged with the responsibility of transporting my mother to the psychiatric division of New York Hospital, which is located, fortunately, not far from where we live. I hope that I can make the short trip without incident.

Earlier this afternoon I spoke with Dr. Haycox, Mom's psychiatrist of many years. "She is moaning. Loudly. And rocking back and forth," I tell him in a whisper, so she won't hear me. But I don't think she would comprehend my conversation anyway.

"Bring her in," he instructs me tersely. There is no denying by the sound of his voice that he is worried. Although I have seen Mom depressed many times in the past, I've never seen her like this before. This is different. It is scary. I wonder why I have been designated to take charge of Mom's deteriorating mental status.

I know that my mother is manic-depressive. She has been like this all of her adult life. Her long depressions are punctuated by shorter periods of something less like happiness and more like jubilation. It's almost as if she has to make up for the time she has lost to depression. Inevitably, though, Mom seems out of control, talking a mile a minute, active all the time, involved in things she cannot even consider when she is depressed.

Her doctor has been advising her for months to try a new drug or combination of drugs. I know she's tried several medications over the years, but none have been effective in getting her out of a depression and preventing her from getting too high. Dr. Haycox has told Mom that in order to effectively monitor her, she will have to be admitted to the psychiatric hospital. But she has no desire to voluntarily commit herself.

What he has suggested, I later learn, is something called an MAOI (monoamine oxidase inhibitor; Nardil is the specific drug), along with lithium. There are risks and dietary restrictions, but he believes that this is her best chance to get the disease under control. What other choice is there? He knows that she has been spiraling downward to depths that he has never witnessed in the years he has treated her. I think that this is what rock bottom must look like.

"In the end, Mom has won her hard-fought battle."

Mom looks over at me as we make our way to the hospital. I believe that a small part of her realizes the significance of what is happening. But it's impossible for her to recognize that my own fragile emotional state is making it more difficult for me to play this role. Later, guilt will set in. I will assume that I must have contributed to Mom's depression by sobbing to her uncontrollably about my life.

Once in Dr. Haycox's office, Mom suddenly begins to scream at the top of her lungs. Looking at her with a level gaze, Dr. Haycox tells her in a controlled voice, "Stop that right now." She complies, crumples into a chair and is quiet. All I want to do is leave. When her husband Bob arrives, I am able to mentally relieve myself of this burden, albeit temporarily. Mom will be admitted this afternoon and remain for three months.

I will visit her only once during that time. I cannot bear to walk through the ward, seeing the vacant stares of the other patients, knowing that Mom is a part of this world. The immature, needy part of me feels completely abandoned by her and by her inability to be the mother I want her to be, need her to be.

There is, however, a bright light on the horizon. Months later when she is discharged, Mom has made a vast improvement. She is still fragile, easing her way back into reality, but she is what others might consider "normal." Mom has weathered this storm. If she continues to stay on these drugs and abide by the dietary restrictions, there's a good chance that she'll be able to avoid the highs and the lows.

Medical science has no cure for bipolar disorder, but it does have an arsenal with which to combat the symptoms. In the end, Mom has won her hard-fought battle. That frightening trip we made on a summer day so long ago did have a happy ending. Mom is back, at last.

Patricia D'Ascoli is an award-winning journalist who writes for a number of publications. Her essay *Choices* was published in *Voices of Breast Cancer.*

Hope

Annie Kassof

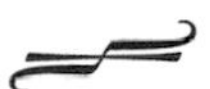

"Give me your hands," I tell sixteen-year-old Justin.

"Here's some of my strength for you," I say. I grasp his hands in mine and look into his faraway eyes. He sits across from me in a vinyl-covered chair. He looks pale and vulnerable in the sunlight that pours through the windows of the psychiatric hospital's visiting room. He's been a patient here for nearly a week, ever since the suicide attempt. His ten year-old sister burst into tears when she heard the news, but I'm still too numb to cry.

The tightness in my chest hasn't gone away since Justin's diagnosis of bipolar disorder, a few days after he was admitted to the hospital. I don't feel strong at all now, but I pretend I do for my family's sake. I'm the only parent they've got. Neither my adopted daughter nor I can comprehend the internal demons of mental illness that led Justin to the precipice between life and death, but obviously we both want him healthy and whole again.

Today, however, my own sanity is feeling dangerously fragile. I *make* myself tell Justin, willing myself to believe it: "Things will get better."

On another day when my daughter wants to visit Justin, too, we arrive at the hospital early enough that she can go to the gift shop, where she buys him a present with her own money. She has the clerk gift wrap it while I sit in the lobby reading a book called *When Someone You Love Has a Mental Illness*. Now, in the visiting room, my daughter leans forward in her chair to watch as her older brother fumbles with the ribbon on the small white box she's just handed him. His hands are trembling—a side effect of the new "cocktail" of medications he's on.

"How can my sensitive, intelligent, vegetarian son be so tortured inside?"

"Open it, Justin," says my daughter, squirming with anticipation.

A few days earlier, as we were buzzed in through the massive metal doors, we heard someone screaming. My daughter stopped in her tracks, clutching my hand. "You don't have to go in if you don't want to," I'd assured her. "It's okay, I want to see Justin," she'd replied. But her brown eyes were frightened as we watched a nurse hurrying the distraught patient out of sight. It wasn't the first time I'd wondered if taking my ten-year-old to visit her brother in the psych ward was the best idea. But after Justin's suicide attempt and unanticipated diagnosis, I didn't want my daughter to feel she was being cast aside as I struggled to grasp the ramifications of my son's illness on our family.

In the sun-filled room, Justin tentatively pulls at the blue ribbon. I force a smile, but inside, unanswered questions fill my mind. How can my sensitive, intelligent, vegetarian son be so tortured inside? Will he be able to return to school? Will he have to be on medication for the rest of his life?

More selfishly I think, when he comes home, will I still be able to find time for my writing career? Will I even feel inspired to write? Will I need to find a therapist for my daughter? For myself? I've been losing weight worrying about these things.

Finally, Justin lifts the lid of the gift box, and nestled in tissue paper is a small, clear stone with the word "Hope" engraved inside. As Justin stares at it blankly without saying anything, I jump from my seat and hug both my kids at the same time, my eyes finally brimming over with tears.

Annie Kassof is a freelance writer living in Berkeley, California. Her stories and essays about her family have appeared in the *Los Angeles Times*, the *San Francisco Chronicle*, *Adoptive Families Magazine*, and many other publications.

Bipolar Disorder: A Mother's Perspective

Jamie Weil

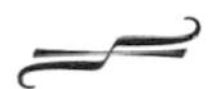

I looked at my newborn baby. She shone back at me. I was 22 years old. We were on our own. I vowed to protect her. How was I to know that voices inside her head would one day tell her to take her own life?

When my daughter, Amanda, was in fourth grade, I was teaching second grade at the same Southern California elementary school she attended. We drove to and from school together every day and often she'd visit my classroom throughout the day. Raising her alone bonded us. We were a team. I felt I knew her very well.

One day the assistant principal called me in to tell me Amanda was having "issues" on the playground. Parents had called and complained. How could I have missed that, being right there with her? I was devastated. I was one of *those* parents that teachers talk about in the staff lounge: the kind who thought they knew their child, but didn't. The school referred us to a local counselor. For a while, things seemed better.

A couple of years later, I retired from teaching to parent a new baby and devote my time to raising the two children. They needed me to be with them, and I had married a wonderful man. Then, as sixth grade began, I was called in to the counselor's office. Amanda had been drawing disturbing pictures of dead people and dripping her blood on her papers. Around the same time, I was noticing odd behaviors at home. There were lots of lies, but what kid doesn't lie? She seemed to hate her parents, but don't they all? She was our oldest child, and we thought this might just be how teens act. She struggled with sleeping, but she had never slept well. She would scream and cry in her sleep and jolt awake. Eyes wide with terror, she was unable to describe the images she saw because they were too horrifying. She would talk about "hating her life" and wanting to end it.

I was crushed; I had failed her. Not knowing what to do, we continued with counseling, and created extra space for one-on-one mom time to keep communication channels open. I wasn't sure what Amanda's problem was or how to fix it, and nobody else seemed to know, either.

As time passed, problems escalated. Counselors referred her to other counselors for comprehensive testing. One well-known psychiatrist introduced us to the terms obsessive compulsive disorder (OCD) and bipolar disorder, and then sent us home with samples of an antidepressant. Half way home, Amanda hung her head out the window and screamed "I want to fly." Part of me thanked God she was not so depressed any more and part of me was terrified we were all going to die. Driving down the freeway while trying to hold a manic child in the car felt like standing on the edge of a high cliff and seeing a tornado coming at you. I've since learned that was her first taste of mania, triggered by the antidepressant in her young, sensitive system.

Desperate attempts to reach the doctor were unsuccessful. Amanda shifted between two shores, one filled with crying and the other made up of heightened, giddy agitation. She peeled off her entire thumb nail until nothing but bloody skin showed. She said she couldn't stop herself. I paced around feeling like I would vomit at any given moment. I felt helpless, powerless.

I wondered if it was safe to sleep or if I should watch her all night. My threats, cries and pleas to the receptionist finally connected me with the doctor after four days. He was on his way out of town and said I'd need to check her into the psych ward at UCLA. How could I check my baby into the psych ward? How could this be happening? She was only eleven years old. I couldn't do it. Instead, my manic child and I set out to find a new counselor and a new psychiatrist, a very disheartening task, as good ones have month-long waiting lists. We knew we could not wait months.

Determination finally landed us in the offices of what Amanda would dub later her "Turn-Around Team," and she would continue with the psychologist and psychiatrist for the next seven years. During this time I read every book I could find on bipolar disorder. She had originally been diagnosed with anxiety and OCD, but I had hunches from researching her symptoms that more was happening. Tapped out by doctor's appointments and a new baby, I would search online late at night for information. I joined the Child Adolescent and Bipolar Foundation and their parent online support group. This was a perfect place to ask questions about new medications, symptoms, doctors and so forth. It was through a parent in that group, not any doctor I ever talked with, that I learned about the National Alliance for the Mentally Ill (NAMI) and the Family-to-Family class, a free twelve-week course for people with mentally ill relatives. I signed up my husband and myself.

"I was one of those parents that teachers talk about in the staff lounge: the kind who thought they knew their child, but didn't."

I struggled with how much to teach Amanda as we went along. After all, she was pretty sure it was me that was "crazy" and would intermittently stop taking her meds by hiding them inside her teddy bear. Talking about mental illness made her feel like damaged goods and she already struggled with low self-esteem. She liked her counselors for the most part, but definitely went through phases when she didn't.

The next phase took us through hell: middle school and high school. Amanda hated me during this phase, which crushed me because I had felt we were so close during her younger years. She hid her involvement with alcohol and drugs, and would lie when we became suspicious. Later in her teen years, we started no-notice drug tests. Failed tests would carry harsh consequences. We needed to learn more than we wanted to know about how long street drugs stay in the system and when to test. We had to become spies and detectives, with our own MySpace page: MomandDadarewatching. We had to deal with teen driving and car crashes. It was an emotional whirlwind and at times I wondered if I could continue to ride.

Amanda's system was extremely sensitive and she seemed to get every side effect from each medication—and we tried them all. Her psychiatrist said she was the most difficult case she had ever had to medicate in 30 years of practice. Some sessions were spent in complete silence with just Amanda and the doctor looking at each other. We also tried every holistic method we could think of, but nothing seemed to give her relief for long.

During this time there were other struggles that frequently accompany bipolar disorder, and some that were just her personal flavor. These included constant suicidal ideation, including one attempt when she was 16, psychotic symptoms, an eighty-pound weight gain which ended her athletic career, street drug abuse, self-injury, panic attacks, stigma from other parents and students, eight crisis hospitalizations, hyper-sexuality and the all-around chaos that comes with Bipolar I with psychotic features, her eventual diagnosis. She had ultra-rapid cycling and mixed states as well, so she would be depressed and manic simultaneously, or moving between poles many times a day. She would cover her ears, scream into a pillow and pound her feet. The tortured look on her face tortured me. I wished I could trade places with her so she wouldn't suffer so much.

Despite the turmoil, we battled hard to keep a sense of humor. We needed one. It was our best tool. Amanda has a highly-developed sense of humor and we look for the funny wherever we can find it. Some may call it a defense mechanism. For us, it is our key to survival. The hardest days are those when we can't find something to laugh about.

Through all this, Amanda managed to keep her grades up and stay active in school. She attended a small high school with small classes which helped tremendously. Extremely creative, she began to show her talent in photography and writing during high school. She used her writing as a tool to her own recovery, journaling while manic, then going back and reading it later. Amanda developed her own systems for checking her balanced states. She began to manage her own medications. She became more receptive to educating herself about her illness. She'd slip and make mistakes, but she would come back around, get back on track, and show perseverance like I have never seen in another human being. She began to see me as an ally again.

College was next on the agenda. What challenges would this bring? Would she be able to remember her medications without missing a day? Would she be able to steer clear of alcohol when it flowed so freely in collegiate settings? Could she handle the stress of the new environment? Some doctors said she should try; others said absolutely not. Amanda's dream had been to go to college, and she insisted on going. My husband and I felt she needed to live her life, but were also fearful of what might happen if she became unstable. We didn't want to lose her.

By the time we had collectively decided Amanda would go, I had become a mental health activist. My husband and I had trained to teach family-to family classes after taking the class ourselves. We began teaching other families and supporting them in their journeys. I joined the NAMI South Bay board as the Vice President and began attending state and national conferences, as well as multiple mental health conferences around California. I envisioned my purpose in this world as arming people going through this battle with the tools they need to survive and thrive through recovery.

The day Amanda left for college and we handed her a lock box with her meds, I worked out in the garden, filled with both joy and fear of what was to come. I planted about 100 bulbs and was in the back yard for about eight hours. Her suicide attempt had involved taking all her week's meds, and since that time they had been locked and dispensed to her. Now, she was in charge.

Amanda settled into college life at a small, private liberal arts university three hours from home in Southern California. She would live in the dorm her first year, then move out into an apartment her second year. Within weeks, we all knew we had made the right decision. Throughout her four years, there were various struggles as there are with many college students, but Amanda developed a responsibility for managing her own illness and handled problems as they arose, appropriately asking for help when she needed it.

During those four years, Amanda learned to take ownership of her mental illness. She spoke in our Family-to-Family class, leaving all family members that listened inspired and hopeful. She managed her own sobriety from alcohol and street drugs. She realized the turmoil caused by missing her "nerve pills" and stayed faithful to her medication regime with the help of her psychiatrist. She learned to find her own doctors and to be proactive, changing professionals if she felt they were not helping her appropriately.

Today, Amanda is 21 years old. She is learning to break mental illness stigma, despite the risk that revealing her own illness may lead to discrimination against her. She has used her experiences to educate and help others in her community with compassion and understanding.

Amanda is graduating with honors next weekend. In four years, she has earned a B.A. in Women's Studies, was nominated for senior of the year, has won numerous awards and was chosen for *Who's Who in American Colleges and Universities*. She has written numerous winning grants, one of which paid for a camp she arranged and ran for high-risk teens, many of whom have said it was the most meaningful event in their lives. She has involved herself with mental health peer groups that meet regarding Proposition 63 funds, also known as the California "millionaire tax" aimed at funding new mental health programs. This year, we will all be attending the national NAMI conference in San Francisco as a family.

Amanda's mental illness is not who she is, but only one facet of a multi-faceted, multi-talented human being with much to contribute to this world. She has only just begun. I am extremely proud of her perseverance, and as her mother, I am honored to share her journey wherever it leads. I have never met a braver soul. She is my hero. And now she calls just to say, "I love you."

Jamie Weil, the mother of Amanda Weil, whose own story appears on the following pages, is a freelance writer who moved back to her home town of Cottonwood, California after a 26-year stay in Southern California. Prior to relocating to Northern California, she served as the Vice President of South Bay NAMI and taught Family-to-Family classes with her husband. She is currently working on a young adult fiction novel in which the 17 year-old protagonist discovers she has bipolar disorder.

Bipolar Disorder: A Daughter's Perspective

Amanda Weil

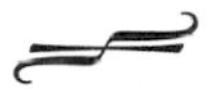

Why was it so loud? Why wouldn't everyone just leave me alone? Why was I so wrong?

Fourth grade marked my entrance into what seemed would be a journey that would only end in death. One night I found myself sitting up in bed listening to the voices that had suddenly erupted in my head. They detailed the plan they had in store for me: suicide.

The voices developed over time, finding a place inside my mind where no other person would be allowed. I began to isolate from anyone who might uncover what was lying beneath my young smile. I began having issues with control, bullying everyone on the playground because it seemed to be the only thing I could manage. My friends became afraid of me, teachers and principals told me it must stop, and my mother, a teacher at my school, seemed lost and terrified.

I learned to hide, lie and manipulate myself out of trouble. This tactic served me well for the next two years or so, until it all became too much to hide. In sixth grade, my younger brother was born and my mother had left teaching to be home. Part of me resented that she was never home for me, but part of me understood that she couldn't be. Though both she and my stepfather tried to reach me, the voices in my head (dominated by one in particular whom I had named Patty) reminded me that they were not to be trusted, that they would foil all of my plans.

I woke up every morning wanting to die. I couldn't stand it, and I developed a self-injury problem. I would cut and pick myself until I found blood. It was an obsession. I knew nobody else that had such a desire and felt further alienated from my friends and family. My thoughts were morbid, clouded with images of death and pain, and I unconsciously began to reveal them to other people. When they displayed concern, I couldn't understand why because in my brain it all made sense. The pain I felt inside was equal to the death I drew on paper.

I never slept. Being tired was the better option to the terror that erupted during slumber. I saw myself committing suicide, and worse, I saw myself killing others. I had no understanding of why and even less understanding of how to stop it. To aid me in my struggle, my mother took referrals from psychiatrists and psychologists. Thus began my trials with medications. From that point until now, I have attempted various combinations of 27 different medications, though it is the first that I will never forget. Eager to test it, my mom handed me the pill in the drug store parking lot. I swallowed. I waited. Suddenly, warmth opened my eyes to the vivid colors that saturated the world. I wanted to dance. I wanted to sing. I wanted to fly. I put my head out the window to feel the air brush my skin and I felt what I had been searching for: freedom.

As fast as freedom had found me, it hid again. Voices teased that I would never be free. What was I thinking? They were right. I fell deeper into the darkness than I had ever been. I knew it now; the voices were right. Ending my life would be the only escape.

I began using drugs and alcohol to find any sanctuary, if only for an instant, from the torment I was battling. Counselor after counselor referred me away. My mother had books detailing various mental illnesses. Diagnoses flew around, eventually landing on early onset bipolar I with psychotic features and obsessive compulsive disorder. They threw in seasonal affective disorder and anxiety, but we had larger issues to deal with. As these dialogues went on I felt more and more insane, broken, diseased and hopeless. Simultaneously, it became easier to tell my parents that I hated them than to tell them that I needed them. I think—or at least I hope—that they always knew the latter was true.

By high school, I had developed a balance between healthy and unhealthy activities. I loved basketball, had plenty of friends, and found that classes were the only place people didn't bother me to talk about my feelings; therefore, I loved being there as well. Concurrently, I found myself drinking and using drugs any time I had the chance, still obsessed with self-injury and engaging in dangerous sexual and social practices. I felt I was living a double life, and though I knew the danger it would lead me to, there was nothing that I could do to stop myself. I developed faulty rationalizations for my behaviors and feelings. I stopped taking my meds when I felt better, started using more drugs and inevitably landed back in the same cycle. Because of the drug use I found myself once again lying.

As it always had, my world came crashing down. It was a Monday morning. I walked downstairs sipping the orange juice that my mother would leave on my dresser each morning before I woke up (to encourage me to take my medicine). I arrived at my per-week pillbox. We filled it together Sunday nights, so it was at capacity. The voices were yelling "Take it, it's time!" I swallowed everything. Every last pill. I drove to school and as I pulled into the parking lot I felt sick. I walked about fifty feet before passing out. I opened my eyes to my mother's frantic screaming:

"What have you done? What have you done?" She didn't wait for an ambulance, but dragged my limp body to the emergency room, crying the whole way.

The next memory I had was opening my eyes to my mother's. She hovered over me in the hospital bed, trying not to cry, and failing miserably. This became the first moment I knew I needed to do something. The voices were strong, but something inside me knew that I was stronger.

> "I opened my eyes to my mother's frantic screaming: 'What have you done? What have you done?'"

From that day on I moved forward and never looked back. Trials with drugs, alcohol, self-injury and my past still plagued me. The factor of addiction was strong, but with the help of various programs it began to subside, and I began to shine again, just as my mother described me as a child.

It came time for college preparation and the furious battle of whether to let me go or not. Many discouraged, many encouraged. My parents asked me how I felt about going, or maybe just taking a year off. As we sat in the afternoon around the dinner table I looked at them both and asked them to trust me, and assured them I could do it. Though I wasn't sure that I could, I knew I needed to change, and college seemed to be the best avenue. To my surprise, they agreed. Their deeper understanding of me, despite all obstacles, has been essential in seeing me through the management of my illness.

Four years later, I am preparing to graduate with honors and move on to the next phase of my life with a stable balance of medication, clean and sober, with a healthy relationship and loving family. I have been very active on my college campus and in my community, engaging young people with similar struggles to those that I have faced. My experience is far from over, but with the balance that I have found, I wake up each morning in search of experience and life and call my family as often as I can, just to say "I love you."

Amanda Weil graduated with a Bachelor of Arts degree in Women's Studies from University of Redlands with honors. While there, she was a campus organizer and activist, served in university government and won numerous awards, including Best Educational Series award for community activism awareness training. She will be listed in the upcoming *Who's Who in American Colleges and Universities*. Her passions revolve around non-profit work and grassroots activism. She recently moved to San Francisco, California to begin the next chapter of her life.

Research Takes Brains

Judith Beth Cohen

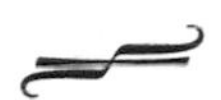

"What is it?" Mother asked. I was visiting her in the day room of the psychiatric unit, where she'd been for over a month.

"A support group for patients and their families," I explained. "I think we should go." Her manic phase long past, she spent most days lying inert in bed. For the past twenty years she'd been in and out of so many hospitals I'd lost count. After my father died, I was the person summoned whenever she cycled downward. I'd fly across the country to visit her and consult with her doctors. And here I was.

"I can't wait to get out of this place—the food is terrible," she said.

She'd lost so much weight that her size ten slacks looked roomy enough to accommodate both our bodies. At least she'd stopped complaining that someone was trying to poison her.

"So, how about that meeting? The nurse thought it would do us both some good."

"Which nurse, the fat one? That slob with the dyed red hair? Don't believe a word she says." Mother headed back to her room and plopped down on the bed.

"I'm going," I said. "I've come a long way to visit; I think you could try, for my sake." Moving in slow motion, she sat up, slippered her feet and followed me to the elevator.

We were warmly greeted by volunteers sitting under the MDDA banner: the acronym for Manic Depressives and Depressives Association, an organization founded and run by people with the same condition mother had been suffering from for most of her life. Here were Our People—hundreds of them it seemed, greeting each other, perusing books and pamphlets on everything from psychopharmacology to filing for disability benefits. How amazing to discover that we weren't outcasts, alone in our deviance, but part of a mass movement.

"Look, Mother," I said. "All of these people have the same problem. Isn't that something?" But the surge of hope I felt didn't seem to reach her.

The greeter explained that after the speaker, we could attend "sharing and caring" groups run by volunteers. We should go to the Newcomers Group, but after tonight we would have our choice: Family and Friends, Women's, Teens, Manic, Depressed, or Bipolar. Mother could have fit several of these categories.

We found seats and I explained the evening's format while a woman lugging two heavy medical volumes joined us. She introduced herself and cheerfully filled us in on her own bipolar disorder.

"For a whole year I had to give up pizza. You can't have cheese if you take MAO inhibitors. Then I took myself off the drug and ate as many pizzas as I wanted and felt instantly better."

My mother looked at her as if she'd just arrived from another planet. The woman went on, offering to look up Mother's drugs in her book, but neither of us could remember their names. The featured speaker, Dr. Crain, an upbeat, energetic young woman with a long braid hanging over her shoulder, looked more like a milkmaid than a neurologist.

"We get seventy brains a year from people with Huntington's Disease, seventy! And there are less than a thousand cases per year in the U.S. Compared to that, 10% of the population has a serious mental illness, but they rarely leave their brains to research." The brain bank she worked for had a twenty-four hour hotline, and she urged us to consider donating.

"My mother laughed, just a short blip, but the first sign that her mood was about to shift."

"I don't believe this," Mother fidgeted next to me.

"Think of it as helping science, your contribution to posterity," I said.

To my amazement, my mother actually laughed, just a short blip, but surely the first sign that her mood was about to shift.

"Don't you know it's against my religion?" she said.

"What is?"

"Jews don't give their body parts away; it's a sin. Didn't they teach you that in Sunday school?"

"I don't remember that lesson," I said.

She refused to stay for the discussion groups, and I took a bumper sticker from the display table as we left. In white letters against a red background, it read: "Research Takes Brains," followed by an 800 number. Suddenly, a tune popped into my head and I couldn't stop myself from singing the lines as they came to me:

> "In my heart, I was thinking,
> I could be another Lincoln,
> If I only had a brain."

"Isn't that from The Wizard of Oz?" Mother asked.

"Yes," I said, pleased that she recognized it, "the Scarecrow's song, remember?"

"Whatever made you think of that?" Mother said. She smiled at me as if we'd just shared a private joke. If she kept this improvement up, she'd soon be released and I could fly home. I escorted her to her room, gave her a hug and rushed back in time to catch the last half of Share and Care.

Judith Beth Cohen is a writer and teacher whose work has appeared in *Women's Review of Books*, *Rosebud*, and the *Mochila Review*. Her novel, *Seasons*, is available from The Permanent Press.

Committal

Anne Skal

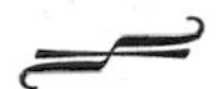

"Your little boy is just fine, Mother," the elderly psychiatrist said, patting my arm, after an hour-long initial session.

How could our six-year-old be "just fine" when for the past three years his moods were like hills and valleys? A few days of very happy, jump-from-the-porch type of activity to several days of rages and anger.

A week later, we received the written report. As we suspected, Michael was not "just fine." Michael had the symptoms of bipolar disorder, once known as manic-depression. But since our son was only six, we chose not to administer any medication nor take him back to that doctor, who told me he was "just fine" yet wrote a report that was totally different. Instead, my husband and I adjusted his diet, read numerous books, and consulted with the school's child study team.

When Michael was eleven, the true downhill spiral began, and one evening I found myself with my son in the psychiatric emergency room at our local hospital.

The fluorescent lights were harsh in that area, hidden away from the "regular" emergency room. The only access was through a key-pad-locked steel door. I sat on a blue plastic chair, hugging myself, feeling so cold despite the heavy winter coat I wore.

My child's voice called from the cubicle nearby. "Mom." Just that. "Mom." Simple, short, plaintive. My whole body ached to rush over to him, hold him, hug him, take him away. I was supposed to be the protector, instead I feel like the instigator.

"We gave him a shot of Ativan, ma'am. He's getting groggy, which is good." The nurse stood several feet away from me, her arms defensively crossed. The security officer was nearby, on call for dangerous people like my slightly built four-foot, eight–inch son, the only patient there.

People told me he looked like an angel, with his dark curls and long dark lashes. But I knew his cherubic face could turn into a rubbery façade when a rage broke through, like that day. Hurtled verbiage spat out at my unconditional love in the safety of our home; objects turned dangerous at the slightest provocation.

"Someday, I thought, he will understand that what I did by committing him was done out of love."

He had picked up a large wooden chair that afternoon, brandishing it like a lion tamer. Only he wasn't play-acting. He was raging. I watched, mesmerized, by the way his face contorted, fearful of what could come next.

My hand reached out to his. "We need to get dinner ready now," I lied. "We're hungry." I had to be very careful with my wording. He usually reacted positively to "we." "I" was too personal, too unforgiving.

He threw the chair across the room, past me. I heard a crack but didn't turn around. I kept my eyes on him.

"Help us call 911," I said more calmly than I felt, edging my hand behind me, along the counter to the portable phone. He came to me then and held fast, as if we were together on a roller coaster ride, waiting for that last, sharp, stomach-turning drop.

Dinner hour was spent in the psychiatric emergency room. I should have been hungry, but I knew if I were to place even a piece of spearmint gum from my purse into my mouth, I'd throw it up. I sat alone, tears burning my eyes and my hands twisting in my lap. Soon I would have to sign the papers to commit my son to a psychiatric facility for children.

A few hours later, in the quiet darkness of night, Michael was transported by ambulance to another hospital a hundred miles away. I rode in the front seat, feeling as if it was all a bad dream. The ride was bumpy, the ambulance sterile and cold. The journey took us through a sleepy town nestled on a hillside. As we wound our way to the top, I looked up and saw an imposing old Tudor-style building; to my tired mind it looked like a fortress. This was where he will stay, I wearily thought. This is where I will leave him.

I said goodbye to my son as they carried him off on the stretcher to his room. He was asleep in a world of happiness and comfort, which at that time was the best place for him to be. For me, I had to face reality with tears in my eyes. At that moment, I felt all alone and wished to fall in a heap on the floor, instead I gathered up whatever courage and strength I could muster and climbed back into the ambulance for the long ride home.

Finally, at one in the morning, I curled up in bed under the warmth of my down comforter, the reading light punctuating the darkness. I could not sleep; I could not understand how my husband, or in fact the rest of the world, could sleep while I felt so restless, so disturbed, and so alone.

Minutes, hours, days, crawled by; voices and faces hovered on the perimeter of my consciousness, soon to be forgotten. I anticipated visiting day with longing, but when the time came it was more disturbing than not seeing my Michael at all. My son stood before us, irritated and upset. The leave-taking was worse than the visit. Recriminations, promises, begging, and finally, anger at being left behind. His childish voice echoed and bounced off the soothing blue walls as we left, my husband pulling me along.

"You needed to do this," he whispered in my ear, hugging me close.

I looked back. The large arm of a male nurse crossed my child's chest, holding him, making sure he stayed within that room. The forlorn look on Michael's face stays within my heart.

I knew that in seven days I would be able to bring him home. There would be medications that he desperately needed, a new therapeutic regime, and mostly new hope. Someday, I thought, he will understand that what I did by committing him was done out of love.

It is a decade later, and improvements in meds and a wonderful and knowledgeable psychiatrist have helped our son become the fine young man he is now. He still has times when he needs to be admitted for inpatient psychiatric care, for "tune-ups" (as he calls them), but it's no longer as agonizing to him or to us. As with most illnesses, he's watchful and realizes that it's something he has to live with for the rest of his life, but he does not allow it to define him.

He is our son. He is Michael.

Anne Skal is a freelance writer with several essays, short stories, and poems published in magazines and newspapers.

PART FOUR

"...none of us understood my wife's disorder..."

"...my husband deserved my help and support..."

"...we are *the caregivers*."

Almost Contagious

Caroline Nye

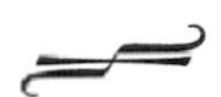

I tiptoed into the bedroom of the elderly man I had been caring for on and off now for several years. It was still quite dark outside, but I opened the curtains anyway, gently tugging them back so as not to awaken Albert too suddenly. He was hidden under the crumpled white sheets, his head covered as it usually was: hiding from a world that was progressively difficult for him and those closest to him. I wondered if there was some way to wake him that wouldn't startle him and propel us all down the road to another dreadful day. I knew deep down that there wasn't.

I was sent to Albert several years previously to look after him as a live-in caregiver. He was having trouble walking due to a severe case of lumbar arthritis and he was suffering from some confusion, forgetting when to take his pills, or remembering twice and overdosing. Apart from these symptoms, he seemed a very intelligent, normal gentleman, with a fascinating history of fighting in the Second World War. Maybe I didn't notice any other symptoms, maybe there weren't any as of yet.

Albert was diagnosed a year later with having bipolar affective disorder. I returned to care for him and initially I couldn't notice any change. Then one morning, his behavior seemed extraordinarily different. His mood was incredibly agitated and he became angry at the smallest of details. His temper became progressively worse as the day went on, and I realized he was having an episode. Suddenly, the enjoyable, peaceful weeks became strenuous and frustrating. Living with Albert day in and day out made me feel as if I was gradually contracting the disorder myself.

Over the coming weeks, I found that Albert's bipolar could seem like a contagious illness: it could seep through mental boundaries and transfer itself to others. I lived and worked with Albert for 22 hours each day, and was astonished at how much his illness could affect those around him. I watched family members come in for day-long visits and walk away in much the same mood that Albert had been in for that day. Sometimes they'd practically skip out of the door, singing happily. Other times a black cloud hung over them and they would be muttering angrily under their breath as they took their leave.

Albert's pride forbade him from admitting that there was anything wrong. The words "bipolar" and "episodes" were met with denial, and the even stronger "mental illness" with anger and some confusion. After a prosperous career and having been a deeply respected gentleman all his life, Albert simply couldn't come to terms with an illness that was out of his control and understanding.

The sharply changing behavior continued and the illness manifested itself in many ways while the correct dosage of medication was slowly being fine-tuned. Sometimes he would be out of control. And then, as if somebody had wandered past and nonchalantly flicked a switch, Albert's behavior would return to normal. These periods of normalcy could last for such a time that the existence his bipolar almost seemed like a dream, a strange memory that held no comparison to the charm and ease with which Albert greeted his everyday life.

It was always a shock when an episode began again. Sometimes I would find Albert sitting in a corner with his head in his hands.

When I touched him gently and asked if everything was alright, he would look at me with a confused expression and reply, "I am depressed. I don't want to carry this depression about the house with me, so I shall sit here until I can think it away."

I wanted to take his hand and explain why he was feeling depressed, tell him that it wasn't his fault and that eventually the depression would pass. But I had tried before and knew that adding this information to his confusion could somehow make it all worse. Albert always preferred to put it down to having just another bad day.

> "Living with Albert day in and day out made me feel as if I was gradually contracting the disorder myself."

But there were many good days, too, when he would rush about the house, singing at the top of his lungs and trying to get everything done in as short a time as possible. He would exercise fanatically and whip his 90-year old body about the garden as if he were 50 years younger. These days were exhausting for everybody, but they were manageable. His frenetic mood would stir us all into a frenzy of action, and we would end the day exhausted.

But we got through it, and we still get through it. We've found that acceptance on the part of all concerned—Albert, his family and his caregivers—is essential. It has been terribly difficult at times, but Albert has managed to lead a full and satisfying life in spite of it all. His specialist identified the exact dosage of medication to control Albert's mood without inhibiting his personality. This is of great importance to Albert, as he worries that the drugs could mean he "would no longer be me." But the drugs aren't enough. A strong shield of support, love and understanding from those around him not only gives him a sense of safety, but also gives him a real desire to control himself for others' sake.

Although there are still recurrences of dramatic mood swings, they are much fewer and further between than in the first few years. So the "invisibly contagious" disorder has silently retreated from Albert's family and me, allowing us to provide the much needed support and love he has never demanded but always deserved.

Caroline Nye has traveled and worked all over the world, working in organic farming, wildlife guiding, teaching, caregiving, and musical performance, as well as volunteering in various international development projects. She has had articles and short stories published in *Amateur Photographer (UK)*, *Matador Travel*, *Transitions Abroad* and The Healing Project book series, and recently won a Bunac Green Cheese scholarship for humorous writing. Caroline is currently managing a dance team in Spain.

Husband's Two Cents

Jeff McKinstry

Dee and I first met through a mutual friend. She was recovering from a breakdown after leaving her husband, whose bad choices and lifestyle had left the family homeless more than once. I saw through the troubles she was having, and recognized her inner strength and beauty. Removed from her toxic environment, Dee began to emerge as a charming and fun-loving woman. It was the closest to love at first sight that I have ever felt. After dating for a couple months, she moved in with me and a few months later we were engaged.

Her bipolar disorder has been challenging, but we have made it through. Dee's disorder is complicated by her troubled past and by the fact that she has a variant of the illness known as rapid cycling, which can cause a frequently occurring, unpredictable range of emotions. The most important thing I've learned about dealing with this illness is the need to consistently act as one's own advocate, and to stick closely to the routines and treatments that help. For someone with bipolar disorder, what may seem like common sense to others can be very difficult to grasp. The illness often leads to thoughts that may not always be in the best interest of the person who is sick. For example, when Dee's medications are working very well, or conversely, if they are not, she has been tempted to stop using them.

Shortly after our children were born, Dee attempted this course of action and needed to be hospitalized within days, as her mood rapidly elevated to a manic state. Her hospitalization was a very difficult time for me. Functioning as sole provider, single father, and supportive husband was no easy task. The sense of isolation was made greater by the fact that our friends, unable to deal with Dee's illness, disappeared. Even family ties were temporarily strained as we came to grips with the illness.

"Bipolar disorder is a disorder—just that—and you should not let it define you."

Another thing Dee and I found was that it can be all too tempting to just accept a doctor's opinion, even when our intuition tells us that no one in the world knows better how we feel than we do. A good example of this arose when Dee was being treated by a doctor who was regarded as one of the area's leading pharmacological psychiatrists. In hindsight I don't think he ever really recognized Dee's condition. The laundry list of meds he had prescribed left her exhausted and sleeping 17 hours a day, and for the few hours she was awake, she was sullen and unemotional. When I brought this to the doctor's attention, he commented that since she was neither suicidal nor manic to the point of needing hospitalization, he felt her condition was satisfactory. I had to push hard for a less aggressive treatment regimen before the doctor would even consider it.

I made many mistakes in how I dealt with friends and family in that difficult time. None of us understood the disorder, and I couldn't understand how they couldn't understand my unwavering support for my wife. In retrospect, the most important lesson I learned at that time was how essential it is to maintain good communication with both your loved ones and your doctors. Expressing your fears and concerns to both, allowing them to recognize what you are going through, and taking the time to recognize and acknowledge their fears and concerns as well, keeps crucial lines of communication open.

Changes in insurance coverage and requirements have been a mixed blessing over the years. Before her illness was under control, Dee suffered mood swings and behavior that required her to spend about a month each year in the hospital and, as a result, my insurance company labeled her PMI (Persistently Mentally Ill) and discontinued her coverage. Her psychiatrist wasted no time in ceasing services and pointed us to the community mental health system. To our surprise, this was possibly the best thing that could have happened to her. Her moving from being the least functional patient of a noted psychiatrist, who was used to dealing with mildly depressed suburban housewives, to being a relatively functional patient among the more severely disturbed, allowed her new doctors to find a course of treatment that was very effective for her. Previously, the anti-depressants and mood elevators tended to have a "rubber band" effect on her moods, leading to frequent changes in medication and more frustration. Her new doctor found a different drug combination that has led to over a decade of relative stability.

The downside of the community mental health system, in our area at least, is the constant turnover of providers. Although the young residents who rotated through the program were all quite capable from a medical perspective, from a therapeutic perspective there was a severe disconnect. Imagine how difficult it is to establish a bond of trust and understanding with a therapist who has a full caseload and works with a patient for less than a year before moving on to a new assignment.

A relatively recent change with my employer's insurance plan changed Dee's coverage again. This change has allowed her to establish a lasting relationship with a psychiatrist and therapist. She has been able to build trust and make more therapeutic progress than in previous years. This trust has gone a long way towards relieving our emotional pressure and we can look to the future with a little more confidence.

After all these years and all of our experiences, perhaps the best advice I can share is to remind yourself that bipolar disorder is a disorder—just that—and that you should not let it define you. After all, have you ever heard anyone say, "I am high blood pressure" or "I am diabetes?"

Jeff and Dee McKinstry have been married for nearly 20 years and have two wonderful children. Jeff works in the learning organization for a large bank and performs standup comedy on occasion.

Just a Normal Girl

Richard Day Gore

Tap-tap-tap.

The metal tip of my umbrella telegraphs my nervous tension into the sidewalk next to my feet as I stand at a pay phone a few blocks from our apartment, talking with Joy.

Tap-tap-tap. Tap-tap-*tap*.

Joy is bipolar. She's having a manic episode, the fifth she's had in as many weeks. I fled the apartment into a frigid December rain to avoid being hopelessly looped into the endless, swirling illogical logic that spills from her when she's cycling high. Now the storm has passed, at least for a few moments, while Joy is still raging in our kitchen. It's exhausting, to say the least. Last week, her mania was triggered by her finding an overdue bill on the kitchen counter, and it didn't even stop for bathroom breaks for a full 36 hours. She came close to getting violent. This bout would surpass that in about 45 minutes, and it seems as if it might do so, as Joy's voice carries me through a broiling stew of rage and apology, anguish and attack.

Tap-tap-tap.

I keep hoping that when the mania stops, we'll be able to return to the bliss of the early days of our relationship, before the bipolar cat clawed itself out of the bag. Diana, a friend of mine whose mother is bipolar, told me that once the cat is out, it doesn't go back in. That having witnessed the ugly side, you become a perpetual reminder, the very embodiment of stigma, simply because you *know*. You become the enemy.

It feels like that sometimes. It's as if when Joy is calm—her normal self—the Other is lurking just beneath the surface of her eyes, examining me for the slightest hint that can be interpreted as an attack. The carefree conversations we enjoyed months ago are gone now, as I habitually examine each word before allowing it to leave my mouth, scouring possible offense from my speech. Unfortunately, there's one thing I've learned the hard way countless times in the last year: to the Other, everything can be interpreted as an attack. And it frequently is.

That I love Joy is the ultimate complication. Diana says I should either pack Joy's things and take her back to her old apartment in the city, or take myself there. That my life is hard enough. But that's a dreadful thought. Joy stuck by me when I was going through the tail end of an adventure with cancer. She showed strength and determination beyond anyone I'd ever met when she helped me up and down the stairs, cooked healthy meals for me on a very slim budget, worked hard and came home with a smile. It would be flat-out wrong for me to toss her because of an illness.

And I don't care what some people say—it is an illness, not some shameful weakness that makes Joy do "bad" things. Expecting her to be able to control her behavior, or to hold her in judgment for her harsh words and sometimes harsher actions, is simply unfair. It would be like penalizing someone with a broken ankle for not being able to run a race. I know the sweet, good-natured Joy that shares her slender frame with the Other. That's the person I fell in love with. That's the real Joy. That's the person my parents adore, whom my friends are eager to invite into their lives. For them, the cat's still mercifully in the bag.

Only Diana knows, and she didn't find out until a few months ago—after I'd been living in the pressure cooker for a long time. She'd been away at school for the early part of my relationship with Joy. She would listen patiently as I interrupted her studies with late night phone calls to sing Joy's praises. When the Other roared to the surface, I didn't have the heart to tell her. The idea was embarrassing, frightening. I didn't want anyone to judge Joy. I still don't. She's had to eat a boatload of that since her teen years because of her "bad" behavior. I don't want anyone to imply I'm making a "mistake" by loving Joy. Our love, like her illness, is a pre-existing condition.

"Our love, like her illness, is a pre-existing condition."

On break from school, Diana came through town. When she stepped off the bus, her first words were, "Jesus Christ, you've gone gray!" She grabbed my chin and turned me to face my reflection in the window of the bus terminal. The person who blinked back at me was a haggard shell of the man who had said goodbye to her months before. Diana looked at me, concern on her face. I was sure she was going to tell me she was worried about my cancer coming back. But instead she said, "Joy's bipolar, isn't she." That's when she told me about her mother. She'd recognized a fellow veteran. We caregivers have the "thousand-yard stare" of someone caught in the perpetual act of scanning the horizon for deadly ambush.

Tap-tap-tap.

Joy's crying now, the inconsolable weeping of a little girl, which always sounds so jarring because it's in the voice of a capable, 26 year-old professional. No amount of my telling her I love her, that we'll find a way to deal with this, can breech her wall of confusion. Joy begs me to come back to the apartment, that it's going to rain again, I should get inside, that she'll be fine when I get back. I want to believe she'll be fine. In fact, she may be. But for how long?

Joy hears the hesitation in my voice and, as the sky opens up, the tears redouble. She cries the same thing she cried last week, as she dragged herself across the kitchen floor on her knees, clutching her hands and beseeching:

"I'm just a normal girl... *I'm just a normal girl...*"

Yes, she is. And no, she's not. It's truly heartbreaking. How could I turn my back on a wound so deep? But I'm starting to feel guilty for worrying about my own well being when it's Joy who suffers with this debilitating illness. The guilt only compounds the internal pressure, because it blurs the lines between so many emotions.

I hoist the umbrella to ward off the pelting rain as I head back to the apartment, but it won't open. It's been utterly destroyed by my nervous tapping: the shaft is bent, the frayed fabric flaps in the cold, wet wind. A car drives past and I catch a glimpse of myself in its windows—a graying man, shoulders low, his being etched with the harsh experience of someone twice his age, dissolved from within by a constant surge of adrenalin.

My mind starts to spin as I anticipate the potential storm that waits in my home, perhaps another 36 hours of operatic mania, perhaps worse. The next level will be blood, I know it.

But perhaps nothing. And anything, and everything, in between.

If I'm not careful, I think as I near the apartment, Joy's illness will drive me insane, too. Take me right down with it. Then up. Then down again. I have to let my own cat out of the bag somehow before it's too late. The two-edged sword of caring for her while caring about her is already carving me up so badly.

But what about Joy? If this is how bipolar makes me feel, the terrible things it must be doing to her are unimaginable.

Richard Day Gore is Senior Editor at LaChance Publishing.

Making Memories

Lisa Fisk

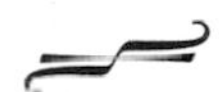

It was early on Saturday morning and the house smelled like burning bacon, fresh coffee, and pancakes. I liked to sleep late on Saturdays. I saw it as my right for having worked hard all week. He, on the other hand, was an early bird; his reward was going to bed while the sun was still in the sky. In the things we both wanted out of life, my brother and I were much the same, but how we went about getting there differed incredibly.

I left my bedroom and staggered down the hall to the kitchen. I found him leaning against the counter, arms crossed in front of him, staring straight at me. This usually wasn't a good sign. Normally the stare-down happened before the big lie. That lie?

"I'm fine. Really."

If you think about it, it's a fantastic lie. Everyone tells it. It's short and easy to remember. Three or four words and the whole world leaves you alone. "I'm fine. Really." Magic under the right circumstances.

Was he fine? Was I? No, not really. I knew what was wrong. I also knew neither of us would ever give voice to how "un-fine" he actually was. Not to each other. We never did: to give *it* a face and a name would give it life, power and control. So we denied the reality of his bipolar disorder until the end.

I copped out after his first suicide attempt; I tried to make him my parents' responsibility. I found myself arguing with them about his treatment and his medications all the time. I never did reject my need to be heard or be responsible for him. Because I already had so many treatment-related conflicts and issues with him, for him, about him, I didn't want to argue with him. I just wanted to love him. We all did.

Today they'd say there was something wrong with his brain chemistry and call him bipolar. Back when he first got sick, they called it "scattered thoughts" or "noisy brain." The medications only worked for a few months, and then he'd develop a tolerance and he'd have to start all over again, or he would deny the illness until it took over and made him uncontrollable. As a family, we all prayed that the next drug would work longer, better, more dependably. Someday, maybe with a little luck, our prayers would be answered. Someday wasn't coming fast enough for any of us.

And what, I wondered was wrong with me? Him. He was wrong and there was no fixing him. I had tried to fix him since the day he came home from the hospital as an infant when I was five. I fixed his diapers, his boo-boos, his little hurts; older sisters are just that way. He came home from the hospital several more times—once for his tonsils, another for the appendix and several times for his busy, creative brain.

"...it changed my perception of reality, of God, of medicine, of life."

That Saturday morning, I silently dared him to look me in the eye. He didn't. He wouldn't. He couldn't. He never could before he lied to me. Instead, he looked me squarely in the nose and concentrated. Most people can't tell when they're being looked in the nose. But since I was several inches shorter than my brother, I figured it out when we were kids. If I could get him to actually look me in the eyes, he'd tell me the truth about anything, about everything. He'd even tell me about the pain, the drain, the rollercoaster, the lack of control.

But he didn't want to tell anyone about his truth; our shared truth. To tell the truth, to pursue new medicines, to get new treatment meant, to him, that he was flawed or broken. He wanted to be perfect. He never realized he was always perfect to me. Even when he was out of control and cycling way too quickly.

"Well?" I asked. I figured we might as well get it over with and then I could drink some coffee.

"Not now, Lisa. We'll talk about it later. Today is a day for making some memories."

At least by not talking we weren't lying to each other. Not talking isn't the same as lying. There was a lot of silence in the apartment some days when we were home alone together.

"What kind of memories?" I asked.

"Well, that's up to you," he said. "I'd prefer good ones, but I could be a real ass if that would make you happy and then we can make some really bad ones for you to remember in twenty years."

"I'll vote for the good ones," I told him. "There are enough bad ones to last a lifetime." I didn't mean to say it out loud but I knew it was true for both of us.

"What do you want to do?" he asked.

"Let's go to the park and feed the ducks. I just want to hang out," I said. His cycling had been rampant and he was about to leave for college, away from adult supervision. I didn't want to do anything that might exacerbate his fragile mood. Had I known that would be the last time I'd ever spend alone with him, I would have chosen something exotic or taken a lot of pictures. I would have done something momentous. I would have picked something so much more significant. I do know that I told him I loved him.

To say that his suicide destroyed my life and that of my family is overstating things. Yes, it was the saddest, most difficult thing I've ever experienced. Yes, it changed my perception of reality, of God, of medicine, of life.

But his death also gave me peace. He hadn't had a quiet moment in his head since he was thirteen. He had to fight constantly to feel what the rest of the world would describe as normal. Now the fight is ours. We picked up his mantle, his battles, and made them our own. It is my hope that one day there will be no more struggles with the pain and chemicals and stigma associated with bipolar disorder. It is my hope that the stigma will end for us all. And that we can all find some peace.

Lisa Fisk is a freelance writer and editor in Phoenix, Arizona. She is an active volunteer for Hospice of the Valley and a former member of the Arizona Suicide Prevention Speakers Coalition.

Hand in Hand with a Bipolar Husband

Maria Sosh

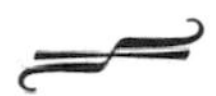

Falling in love is one of those quirks of life that is never expected, always anticipated, and full of discoveries, about the person you've fallen in love with and about yourself. Some of those discoveries bring the chance of shared passions, such as favorite foods, movies, books, and travel destinations. Others reveal the differences that allow you both to be more balanced and fulfilled people when you're together. And then, sometimes, you make discoveries you couldn't have imagined—startling, troubling discoveries that can challenge you, your mate and your relationship.

My first husband and I had lived together for several months, learning that we shared many more passions, especially music and a similar sense of humor, than we shared differences. We took great comfort in that knowledge. But before the end of our first year, my husband began to change. He started having difficulty sleeping, was irritable, and expressed sincere concerns about neighbors watching us. At the time, I tied the irritability and mild paranoia to his lack of sleep.

Over the next year, however, his behavior became more extreme. He developed an explosive temper, would often not sleep for two days, and openly accused me, and others, of devious actions against him. Slowly, over the course of two to three years, my husband went from an open, joyful, talented musician to a brooding young man with dark thoughts, terrible nightmares, and a violent temper. The overall transformation was so slow that my reaction was most often to blame myself for his outbursts, to try every sleep aid possible, and to mold my life around his needs in order to avoid disrupting his seemingly fragile world.

The first doctor we visited diagnosed him as manic depressive and prescribed massive doses of lithium. This treatment never altered the mental and physical agonies my husband experienced, but no doctor offered any other relief. We discovered that enduring a chemical imbalance was a battle we would mostly have to fight on our own, and slowly, but surely, we found small weapons to help in the battle to maintain an essential stability in our lives.

The greatest tool of all was one that may seem at odds with someone suffering from a bipolar disorder, but it worked every time: humor. The ability to laugh saved us one night, after we had both been awake for over 72 hours because of his manic obsessions. He exploded into a rage, grabbed a kitchen chair, smashed it to pieces, and holding one jagged chair leg, struck a threatening posture at me, apparently preparing to attack. At that moment, my mind seemed to sheer away from the reality and suddenly the entire event seemed monumentally absurd. Without a thought, I began to laugh loud and hard. Then I leapt in front of him and assumed an exaggerated samurai warrior pose, grunting loudly and still laughing.

The effect was magical. My husband looked at me with amazement for a moment, and then grunted back at me. We began moving in a circle, doing a ridiculous parody of samurai warriors preparing for battle. My husband suddenly grinned, then shouted unintelligible words in an oriental accent, bowed to me and pretended to stab himself in the stomach with his chair leg "sword." The violence disappeared completely. We stared into each other's eyes. "I want to die every day," he said, "but I know I can't."

We had hundreds more violent face-offs that were defused when I was able to use humor to reveal the dark absurdity of his actions. My husband was and is an extremely gentle, sensitive man who creates beautiful music and dearly loves animals. He cries openly over the cruelties people perpetrate on others and has stalwart values based on honesty and loyalty. He loves comedy and laughs easily at the silly things that we all should laugh at each day. He holds no grudges and forgives readily.

"...we worked together, using humor and intelligence and love to survive."

I cannot count the number of times I was told to leave him. To save myself. To have a normal life and let him go his own way. If we had discovered two or three years into our relationship that he had an incurable, crippling disease, would I have abandoned him? Just because his illness affected his mind didn't make his suffering less than a disease that strikes the body. He was my husband. He needed my support and help. So we worked together, using humor and intelligence and love to survive the frightening manic episodes and the massive depressions.

Our relationship lasted 19 years. When we finally parted ways it was with tremendous anguish. Since we parted, new drug therapies have been discovered that offer him relief. Taken in combinations, these new medications have helped him find a more stable lifestyle, where sleep rarely eludes him and his paranoia is diminished. He still struggles daily in the battle with own his thoughts, but there are more calm days than days of terror now.

I believe my first husband is the bravest man I've ever known, and it has been an honor to know him.

Maria Sosh has been a freelance writer for 30 years, regularly bringing her life experiences to paper. As an editor, Maria supports novice and seasoned authors in the self-help, business theory/strategy, and young adult sci-fi fields.

PART FIVE

"...I have a special gift to share with the world..."

"...inside us all is a world of good possibilities..."

"...I've learned to manage it."

Dealing with Alternative Cloud Patterns

Kathryn Presley

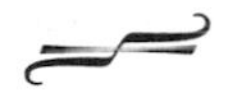

I think of bipolar disorder as "the disorder of being too human." My sickness is that I'm the same as everyone one else, only more so. When the sky turns white, most people pull on their sweaters and sigh and get in their cars and go to work. When the sky turns white, my friends start calling me first thing in the morning to see if I'm okay, if I've gotten out of bed, if I can meet them somewhere just to get me out of the house. After this happens, I pull on a sweater, sigh, and get in the car to go meet one of these friends. Same as everyone else, with a little extra. That's my life as a bipolar person.

It's incredibly easy to think of life pre-bipolar and post-bipolar, but I've learned to stop doing that. I was a weird kid, then a weird teenager, now I'm a weird adult, and I'll be an incredibly weird old lady. Patterns emerge. The difference is, somewhere between adolescent and adult weirdness, I got diagnosed with a mental illness. So did my mother, and so did my sister. And we all freak out when the sky turns white.

I don't regret how I turned out at all. My mom blames herself for passing on this disorder to both of her children, for not having the decency to keep her less desirable genes to herself. I have two arguments against her on this debate. One: If only one child ended up being bipolar, the other child would have been left out of the bonding that would take place between crazy sibling and crazy mom. This would result in all sorts of neuroses that are potentially far less manageable than Too-Humanness. Two: If neither of us had been bipolar, it would have just been Mom, and she would have been lonely. We, her daughters, would not know how to help her when the sky turned white. We probably would have pulled away from her because her mood swings made no sense, her bouts of depression made no sense *and* interfered with getting us to soccer practice, and her bursts of energy poured into work would have just seemed like avoiding time with us. All three of us would have been different people. I wouldn't have liked any of those people.

"I love being so busy that mere mortals cannot keep up with me. I love occasionally staying up all night because my latest idea might save the world."

No, we all got diagnosed, and we all cry too much and laugh too much and sleep too little, and get more done in a hypomanic three days than most people get done in a month. That's not bragging—it's terrifying to have the kind of energy that makes you feel like sleep and food are a waste of time. But it's also sort of rock & roll. And it's like we all have backstage passes to each other's shows, for every stop on every tour. And who wants to come off the best (or worst) show on a sold-out (or totally empty) tour, only to find herself alone on the tour bus (or Dodge minivan)?

Being bipolar is not, by a long shot, easy. I am paralyzed with sadness when the sky is white. I have cried for more than 12 hours straight, gone days without sleep, destroyed relationships, forgotten literally months of my life, acted like an idiot in public, dropped out of school, lost dangerous amounts of weight, and wasted months out of what are supposed to be the best years of my life, lying in bed or staring at walls or asking myself "what if?" I have visualized this disorder as a monster, a cancer, a decay eating its way through the best parts of my brain. I have used it as an excuse for countless offensive behaviors.

Only recently have I started to understand it. Now, for example, I see bipolar disorder as a bumblebee, and I get out of bed just fine. It's a lackadaisical disorder, striking only sometimes, and then only because I was foolish enough to stumble into a place where I knew it lived. Bipolar disorder has territories. It lives late at night in empty houses, dark places that lack natural light. It lives with ex-lovers. If I sit too long anywhere and think purposely of sad things, it will show up and sting me. So lately my exercise is in remembering the places to avoid, which is easier than people tell themselves it is, and I arrive at the beginning of most days sting-free.

I don't ever want to be rid of bipolar disorder. I love being too human. I adore crying, and it doesn't bother me that I cry more often and for longer than most people. It has never failed to calm me down. I love being so busy that mere mortals cannot keep up with me. I love occasionally staying up all night because my latest idea might save the world.

But I am not starry-eyed. This is not an easy disorder to have, and for years I thought it would kill me. I have worked relentlessly and excruciatingly hard to be as healthy as I am. I have changed my diet, gone to counseling, taken medication, and self-reflected enough to give Buddha a run for his money.

I still hate a white sky, and am still too eccentric for many of the people I meet. But I've got my mom and sister, as well as the friends who call to get me out of the house when they know the sky will be white and I'll be having trouble. And I've got a really excellent set of sweaters to choose from before I start even the worst of days.

Kathryn Presley was born and raised in Seattle, Washington. She is currently studying Literature and Gender Studies in Los Angeles.

You Know Me

Pamela Richards

You know me. I'm the small town lady who attends First Baptist Church, singing alto in the choir. I go to Wednesday night prayer meeting and Tuesday morning missionary circle. I'm the woman who smiles politely at strangers and volunteers on the twenty-four hour crisis hot line. I started a jail ministry at Anderson County Detention Center. I lived through integration, when my high school got bombed. I screamed my head off at a Beatles concert, made love not war, and followed Timothy Leary into LSD-land. I lived through a senseless war that took just nine days to steal my fiancé. I went to a major university, married, and birthed three children in two years (twins). I taught English and math in a small Christian school, directed and choreographed a mime group for teenagers, and divorced after twenty years of marriage. I am the woman with gray hair, peering through half-moon reading glasses, looking for the calorie count on the dark chocolate candy bar. I am overweight in denim jeans and jacket, a lost hippie working out at Curves three times a week.

You know me.

And you don't.

You do not know I am bipolar. I cycle from the deep pit of depression to sky-high manias so debilitating that I am on disability for my mental illness. You do not know the generational curse of manic-depression on the women in my family, that my mother died refusing to take her lithium, that my daughter is already on disability for her bipolar at age thirty-two.

You don't know how hard I struggle to be able to lead a valuable, worthwhile life. You do not know about the fourteen hospitalizations, five suicide attempts and my erratic history with medications that resulted in my having to live in a group home for six months. You do not know about the shock treatment that resulted in only six months of stability. You cannot see me in a transitional house with food stamps my only income because the depression is so bad I can't get out of bed to go to my job as a night auditor.

You do not know the multitude of medications I have downed in an effort to control the mania that consequently causes me to cut, burn, shoplift, write bad checks, and go bankrupt. You do not know I have been in therapy for twenty years, or the months I spent in bed, getting out only for doctor's appointments. You have not coped with my extreme mood swings—the highs that keep people hovering at a distance, or the lows that cause them to dress me in black, convinced my death is imminent.

"How did I become the person I am today? Perseverance."

But I have not died; far from it. I am as resilient as an elastic band stretched to the limits of sanity, continually springing back to reality. I have fought my way out of a box of societal stigma and endured a non-existent support system. I welcome you into my world of victory as I grasp life and become the writer I dreamed of being when I was twenty. I write poetry, have finished my first novel, and returned to college at age fifty-six to finish a degree in creative writing, long put aside.

How did I become the person I am today? Perseverance. I accepted the reality that I will cycle again and again like the ebb and flow of the tide. But I now know the pit is not the endless abyss that it seems at the moment, and stability will resurface.

I know you, where you have been, and continue to go. Find the one thing in your life that you can teach others and encourage them. Finally, be gentle to yourself.

Pamela Richards taught English and math at a small Christian school in Virginia and is currently a student at the University of Tennessee, where she is finishing a degree in creative writing. She, her mother and daughter are bipolar.

Forward Momentum

Anne S. Zanoni

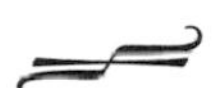

Initially I was a voluntary patient before the merry-go-round known as the mental health system tried to eat me. I checked myself in because I knew I needed a doctor. I was manic, a seemingly helpless passenger in my own body, barely, but sufficiently, able to understand that something was wrong with me.

My first doctor put me on lithium, but my mania didn't change. About three weeks later, I checked myself in to another hospital. There I got pregnant while manic. That doctor never thought to ask whether I was sexually active before he put me on the pill. Nor did he order a blood test, not until I had morning sickness for several days. The doctor watched me when he explained I was pregnant. His hands tightened on his chair in the proverbial death grip, terrified I would insist on keeping the baby, because when you're manic, your judgment is shot. I didn't insist. In spite of my mental state, I understood what fetal mutation meant.

Everything is derailed by rising thoughts: thoughts that explode in your mind and push everything else out of their way. This is what I was thinking then: that a good friend had just had a very bad miscarriage. And, swept up in mania, I considered giving her my just-discovered unborn child the way you'd give someone a kitten.

That rising thought—a mad idea that makes perfect sense to the manic—didn't carry the day.

I have never had children.

Not long after that, my second doctor got a court order to ship me to the state mental hospital. To make me someone else's problem. I'd asked him for another medication, because obviously lithium didn't seem to help. Some drugs do that—they either don't work at all on me, or they work very briefly, and then have no effect. Before that court order, my doctor told me no other drug existed.

"Five years after my first mania, I graduated from college—cum laude."

This was untrue. I have been successfully on Tegretol since mid-1992. The right medication came to me through my next doctor, in what was now my third hospital, about four months after I'd sought medical help. By that point I was firmly stuck in the mental health system as an involuntary patient. Thanks to that court order, I was in a total of four hospitals that year, including the two I checked myself into. Then I went to a Fairweather Lodge, and from there a semi-independent living program.

I got a break in early 1993, because my social worker believed in me. I said I could work. He persuaded the staff to let me, then went even further and got me transferred into a place he felt would suit me better. I went back to the temporary services and working full time. The nice state rehabilitation folks paid for me to finish college, all but my final year. They made me go slowly (unlike that social worker, they didn't believe in my ability to know my own limits) so it took an extra year. But I made it through. Ten years after I graduated from high school, and five years after my first mania, I graduated from college—cum laude.

My third doctor, I think it was, told me that being bipolar was like having diabetes: you take your meds for the rest of your life so you can be well. I heeded him. Unlike many bipolar people, I didn't have to go through many drugs to find the right mix, for which I am profoundly grateful, and I have not been an inpatient since 1992. I have mostly found my own therapists, and I know well the importance of seeing the same therapist who will work with me. Various state health programs gave me a rotation of doctors, but having the same therapist meant I had someone who knew me as her client: a person, not just another patient.

It used to be that when I told people I was bipolar, or manic depressive, invariably the response was, "You're too happy to be depressive!" Of course that has nothing to do with it. Vivacious energy is part of what makes me me and not someone else. But there is something to be said for perseverance. For setting goals. Maybe that's why I checked myself into the hospital years ago. To keep up my forward momentum. I'm glad I did, and I've never stopped.

Anne S. Zanoni is a copy editor who is very active in the Society for Creative Anachronism and science fiction fandom. Her first passion is reading.

Why I Write

David O'Neal

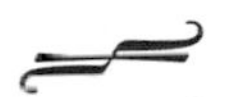

When I was a child, I stuttered so badly that I sometimes couldn't talk at all. Even today, in late middle age, I am fearful of speaking under certain circumstances. Strangely, I speak French, too, and have never stuttered in that language. I think this is because when speaking a foreign language well one assumes a different persona, new and freer, unencumbered by past neuroses. A mask to hide behind. Due to my stuttering, I grew up apprehensive about verbal communication, distrusting speech as a mode of discourse for me. I was very uncomfortable with conversation and began to think oral communication led too easily to misunderstanding. So I learned, and prefer, to express myself in writing. Even in business, I have tried to communicate with clients and colleagues in writing in order to make things clear and to give them time to consider and respond appropriately.

Creative writing is also good therapy, and so it has been to me. I am bipolar (Bipolar II, mostly depressive) and have been hospitalized several times for my own protection when severely depressed. When mired in the swamp of depression, I regress into near infantilism and the old fear of becoming mute becomes nearly realized. While I cannot write during these times of extreme mental stress, at other times creative writing is very good for me. Writing focuses my attention with laser-like precision and forces irrelevant thoughts out of the usual "monkey-mind." In the heat of creating a poem, story, essay—while processing ideas—it is impossible to dwell on much else. Thus, writing sweeps the mind of unpleasant thoughts and has healing power.

Writing is therapeutic and transformational for me in other ways too. It is therapeutic to write about specific personal issues or emotional problems, happy times as well as unhappy—the gamut of emotions and experiences that are heightened by my being bipolar. Such writing doesn't solve the emotional dilemmas written about. Yet, in finally giving these issues full expression, their emotional impact can be pared down and more objectively understood. I can lighten my baggage. Similarly, writing in anger about aggression takes the edge off. Better to write the mystery story than to commit the murder!

"Writing is my shield against madness."

Another reason I write is to impose some sort of order on the occasional chaotic circumstances of my life. Writing is a kind of control, a way to discover meaning in my experience—even to discover wisdom. And to write creatively is sometimes to uncover deeply hidden emotions and ideas not ordinarily accessible to our consciousness. Still another reason to write is to capture, or recapture, memories or incidents worth recalling. It is like taking photographs, but the method is deeper, more reflective, and more analytical.

I am recently retired from the antiquarian book business, during which career I wrote many catalogues offering rare books and manuscripts. I also wrote a number of professional articles about books, libraries and book collecting. Yet I always wanted to have time to write creatively, from the imagination. Now I have that time. Writing takes the time and fills it up—a good thing for someone subject to cycles of despair caused by bipolar disorder. Are not idle hands the Devil's playthings?

While I write essentially for myself, getting my work published offers positive feedback. Attempting to publish takes toughness and moxie, and I feel good that I can go through the process with my sense of self intact. But for me, the bottom line, the reason I write, is always the same: I cannot not write. I have the writing demon that keeps my soul uplifted from deep darkness. Writing is my shield against madness. Writing keeps me sane!

David O'Neal, educated in Switzerland, England and the United States, is a graduate of Princeton, an ex-Marine Corps officer, and a retired antiquarian bookseller who lives in San Francisco with his parrot, Streak. O'Neal's articles, poems, and short stories have been printed in *Sensations Magazine*, *Bird Keeper*, *Marin Poets Anthology*, *The Storyteller*, *The Christian Science Monitor*, *Writers' Circle*, *Writer's Forum*, *Working Writer*, *Street Spirit*, and *Vision Magazine*.

Seeking Freedom

Matthew Rennels

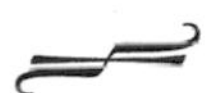

It was the spring of 2007. I stood before the congregation at Restoration House Family Worship Center holding a microphone, trembling. I was about to tell a crowd of roughly eighty people something I hadn't even told eight. I broke into my story slowly, telling them how I went through a mild depression as a college student of 21, a depression that abruptly ended one day when I suddenly became full of life. The next day I felt even more fantastic. The day after that was even better, and so was the next, and the next. I was now full of zest, so much that it began to scare my closest friends and family. I lost my job. I flunked out of school. Things spun out of control to the point that I thought I was Jesus Christ.

At that, the congregation at Restoration house let out a collective gasp. And that's when I found the strength to tell them what I had told so few others:

"My name is Matt, and I suffer from bipolar disorder."

I had guarded those words with my life since 2002, when I'd experienced that brief phase of acute mania. My racing mind was destroying my life, so my parents took me to a psychiatrist, who diagnosed me as bipolar and put me on lithium. I leveled out, but as is common, this was followed by a severe episode of depression.

I'd always seemed like a "normal," happy kid. But all that had changed abruptly, and now I was scared to even leave my home. Speech became difficult. My sentences weren't always coherent. I became deathly afraid of social situations because when words came out, they always came out wrong. I couldn't make eye contact because I was certain people could see into my messed up, disturbed soul. I couldn't see a person without thinking something terrible about them, and I couldn't watch movies or T.V. shows because they would carry my thoughts into very scary places. I often thought about suicide, believing I would probably never return to my old self and that I was only doing everyone a disservice by living. I trudged on, but I felt I had dishonored my family and let down my friends and the community that raised me. I felt helpless as my friendships crumbled and family relations went beyond strained. I had unusual anxieties that made me feel uncomfortable around strangers, but also around my closest friends and my own family.

After sitting out a semester due to academic delinquency, I gave school another try in 2003. It was hard spending so many hours on campus when I was constantly battling anxieties and uncontrollable thoughts that included believing the person next to me in class was thinking about me; focusing on attractive females and thinking they wanted me; being unable to make eye contact with professors; thinking that everybody in the classroom hated me and wanted me to leave, particularly the professors.

It's no surprise that I missed nearly as many classes as I attended, but somehow I was able to graduate with a bachelor's degree in journalism. This graduation day was remarkably different from my high school graduation, which had been a very happy event. This time there were no feelings of accomplishment or excitement for the future, a future that before my depression and mania had included dreams of touring with a successful rock band or becoming a respected music critic. Now, the future held only uncertainty. My ambitions became much more limited: I wanted nothing more than to have a normal, flowing conversation or build a bond with somebody, *anybody*. I wanted people to find out who the real me was, not this shell of a person I had become, and to like me when I was sober, not when I was drunk. But that meant I would have to learn how to speak first.

Speaking was the most challenging aspect of my bipolar experience. Whenever I would start talking, my words would sound weird or dumb, so I would rush through them, and this left the listener confused, frustrated, and sometimes sympathetic. If they were confused or frustrated, I would become even more frustrated and would end the conversation. If they sounded sympathetic, it would hurt my pride because I didn't want pity, and I would end that conversation, too. Obviously, this was quite damaging to my relationships, ending most of them.

Unfortunately, there was one "medicine" that allowed me to at least feel like I was socializing: alcohol. Not a good mix with lithium. I drank massive amounts of alcohol, heading to the bar three, four, sometimes five times a week. Rather than sip a drink and socialize, I went out to slam seven or eight rum and cokes, to the point of belligerence. I was trying to escape my problems, which was impossible because they were deep within me, and I became an alcoholic in the process, going from being a regular churchgoer to never attending at all.

As happens with alcoholics, the drinking only made my problems worse. I was ruining all my friendships. In my moments of clarity I would mourn my days before the depression, when I had been something of a "friend factory," meeting new people and welcoming them into my life wherever I went. But no matter how hard I tried, it appeared there was nothing I could do about this. There wasn't a day that went by that I didn't cry out in anguish, pleading for normalcy, for my life back. I was agnostic, so I never said a single prayer.

In February, 2004 I packed my things into a U-Haul and left my home town, Charleston, Illinois, for the first time ever. I moved to

Murfreesboro, Tennessee, settling into a townhouse apartment with one of my remaining friends. This was likely the best thing I could have done, because I began to find myself again, and I learned about surviving on my own. My social anxieties were still very much alive and my life was still in pieces, but now it was *my* life. My new life didn't start well, however. My friend and I both worked at Home Depot during the day and went to the bars at night. I continued to drink heavily and eat everything in sight, easily surpassing 200 pounds, and I hit on girls everywhere I went, very unsuccessfully.

I realized that this phase of my life was leading nowhere, so I applied for jobs at newspapers and eventually landed a job in Hopkinsville, Kentucky. This was just where I needed to be. Here I found a fulfilling job that allowed me to really apply myself, and I was away from many of the vices that had pulled me down. But things weren't great yet—my anxieties weakened some, but they were still there, lurking and waiting to burst forth, dominating both my thoughts and my social life. My perspective about people continued to be very negative, and I regularly got into fights with my newspaper's editor. I complained all the time, and when I made mistakes, which happened often, it was anyone else's fault but my own. The experience of bipolar had left me an ugly person.

Sitting next to me at the newspaper was a man named Joe. Joe heard my complaints day in and day out, but he did his best to brush them aside. He likely noticed my strange mannerisms and insufficient social skills, but he put those aside, too, and befriended me. Joe didn't flaunt it, but he was a Christian. In fact, I'm not sure how I even found out, but I know it wasn't when our coworkers and I were telling our drinking stories or planning trips to the bar! He never pushed his church on me, and never asked about my faith, though he mentioned going to church with his wife.

Then, one day, I got an impulse to ask Joe if I could accompany him to that church. I think he almost fell out of his chair, since he knew me as a big drinker with no apparent interest in church, but he agreed.

When Sunday arrived, I was terribly nervous as I waited to go into the church. Here I was, my life having been defined by the anxieties, social awkwardness and inappropriate behavior caused by my bipolar, about to step into the place of quiet decorum. It struck me that my anxieties would quiet whenever I walked into a bar, but now that I was about to walk into a church, they raged inside to the point that I felt they were crawling all over me. But in I stepped. I shook some hands, trying my best to put a smile on my face. The praise band began to play and I stood for worship. I thoroughly enjoyed it, but was afraid to clap my hands or show any other gestures. I was beyond self-conscious at this point. The band finished and the pastor asked us to sit, and then my anxieties worked aggressively to keep my focus off his message. But I felt my head nodding in agreement several times (even though I was very self conscious of that, too!)

> "I was learning that I could trust in God... to give me freedom and comfort."

Afterwards I spoke to the pastor, or at least I tried to. I had the hardest time even pushing out a sentence, but I think I somehow got across the point that I enjoyed his message and the music, and he listened intently and invited me back again the next week.

I didn't miss many Sundays after that. Each and every Sunday morning my alarm clock would go off, triggering my anxieties to wake up and get busy along with me. "Don't get up," they'd say. In the shower, they became louder. "Don't go! Nobody likes you at that church and everyone would be better off if you just stayed home!" Even my car rides to church were a challenge, but I made it week after week.

Six months prior to this, I took myself off lithium. I always struggled with lithium, wondering if bipolar was really my problem or if it was this med, and I wondered if I would return to normal if I went off it. I had always remembered my first psychologist telling me about some bipolar cases who successfully went off of lithium. I often went several days without it, but then I would panic and return to it for fear of a relapse. But finally, after four years of living under a heavy intake of lithium, I took the plunge.

I wouldn't recommend this step to anyone, and I know it's best to make any move like this under the supervision of a doctor. I had always expressed my unhappiness with lithium to my psychiatrists, and I wanted to at least try reducing the dosage, but they always talked me back onto the drug and kept me at the same level. In retrospect, I realize I should have kept looking for a psychiatrist who would actually take the time to listen to me and work with me on reaching my goals.

Regardless, something inside me told me to give it a shot, and so far I am blessed with a life beyond lithium. When I went off it, I didn't feel the rushes of confidence I felt in my manic stage during college; I didn't cycle through grandiose visions and imagine myself to be Jesus Christ again. In fact there was nothing grandiose about my wishes: just to be able to hold successful conversations and make solid eye contact. I never had mood swings, and was never near as irritable or overwhelmingly happy as when I was manic. I kept the medicine bottle in the cabinet just in case, and monitored myself closely. In fact, I was extremely careful because every time I felt even a hint of joy I got scared that I was going manic again.

Months passed and nothing much really changed, for bad or for good. I didn't have any manic episodes at all, but I still had all of the old anxieties. But I had equipped myself with a new set of "medicines" to replace the lithium and the alcohol, to deal with the pitfalls of bipolar disorder and deep anxiety. I was learning that I could trust in God, not liquor, to give me freedom and comfort, and soon I was cured of alcoholism. I was also realizing I didn't need to feel guilt anymore for lustful sins or for messing up friendships. I was forgiven. I began rebuilding my character and my social life. I worked diligently to escape the persona I created when I embodied bipolar disorder—the socially inept drinker—and to rediscover who I really was.

So there I was, "coming clean" to those 80 people at Restoration House Family Worship Center, feeling the weight of my secret being lifted from me as I spoke from my heart without shame about my condition, my actions and my circumstance. Thanks to my friend Joe, the welcome of the congregation and, yes, my own determination to lead a better life, I knew I was stepping onto a new path, a path that led both into a better future and back to the happier days I knew before that fateful semester of college, when my world turned upside down.

Since then I have talked to other groups about my battle with bipolar disorder, and I have opened up to the world that I was diagnosed with it in 2002. Today it is my new life direction to help people realize there is freedom from this. I haven't taken any medicine in three years and my abnormal anxieties are finally gone. I met a beautiful woman two years ago and we are getting married in August, and I again have a busy social life. Alcohol, anxiety, mania and depression are no longer the center of my attention. God is.

Matthew Rennels is a 28-year-old writer born and raised in the small Midwestern town of Charleston, Illinois. He recently married a beautiful woman, Tasha, and is living in Clarksville, Tennessee, where he is writing books and working to help people battling depression and anxiety.

Let the Music Be Your Master

Sherry Stearn

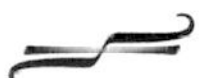

There's a Led Zeppelin song with lyrics that go, "Let the music be your master, will you heed the master's call..." Thanks to my bipolar disorder, some aspects of my history are like those lyrics come to life.

My early teens were the proverbial rollercoaster ride. I had so much energy that it sometimes felt like I was the rollercoaster. I was the picture of the active high school student: very social, lots of friends, good at sports. I loved track and swimming. They were the perfect outlet for the tremendous amount of energy burning inside me. But in addition to the fun and achievement of my social and sports life, I was plagued with what we called "episodes" about every three months during my high school years. During those periods my excess energy would find other, less positive outlets. Trouble with boys. Trouble concentrating on schoolwork. Trouble managing my feelings. I fell madly in love with a boy who was two years older than me. He was on the football team and quite well-known locally. He drank a lot; the classic partying jock. Associating with him exposed me to alcohol which I quickly found I couldn't handle. With alcohol in my system, my emotions could be triggered by almost anything and there was very little grey area once my mind and heart got churning. I got either extremely happy or terribly upset. There was no middle ground. To others, my behavior would seem very exaggerated, but it made perfect sense to me, and no matter how extreme my reactions, they were always justifiable in my own mind.

One rainy night I was watching MTV, and the music started sending me messages. It was as if there were secret words encoded in the lyrics, or an invisible spirit within the music that was communicating directly to me. I hadn't seen my boyfriend in a few days. I decided I was going to find him and tell him how upset I was about this. So I ran the whole way to where he worked as a lifeguard at a hotel pool—almost a mile from my home—without stopping once. He wasn't working, which was a good thing because I was soaking wet and crying inconsolably. I'm sure I appeared pitiful and, yes, crazy to those around me, but inside my feelings and actions seemed completely logical. I sat by the pool and stared at my reflection in the water. Finally I decided to go to his house. Off I ran again in the pouring rain. By chance he drove past me and stopped to pick me up. I started yelling at him for ignoring me, and when he laughed at me I got even more upset. Soon I became hysterical and he drove me home.

Because of this and other episodes, my parents sought treatment for me; I started taking medication and going to therapy. It helped, at least until my boyfriend decided, not surprisingly, to take someone else to the prom. It would have been hard enough for a teenage girl without a chemical imbalance to handle. But it pushed me over the edge. My emotions and my uncontrollable agitation prompted me to start drinking.

This was a bad, bad mix with my medication, and it led to more trouble. I started hanging out with an older crowd that had wild parties. I learned early on that I was very sensitive to any chemicals that would make the rounds at these parties. Either I passed out or I become the life of the party. Again, no grey area. Then, at one party, someone gave me some laced pot. I ended up hallucinating and having an out-of-body experience. My whole system was thrown even more off balance and I ended up in the hospital.

You could say this was a wakeup call, but waking from such a deep nightmare wasn't easy. I found a new boyfriend, a talented musician who was into meditation, alternative healing and herbs—the healthy ones. I did learn how to balance some of my emotions with meditation and to express my feelings by writing song lyrics. He taught me how to structure songs and work with the music. Structure was what I needed, internally. Making myself sit down and concentrate on a writing project made me stay calm and focused, and it helped me to sort through my jumbled emotions.

The restless energy that had driven me into sports (and trouble) started to find an outlet in creative pursuits such as modeling and acting. Doing photo shoots and acting in films and T.V. was a big help, as if I were portraying all the characters and emotions that were boiling over inside of me. I worked in Philadelphia for a while and then decided to move to New York to pursue the Big Apple's many opportunities.

I moved into a model's apartment and started to pound the pavement in hopes of being "discovered." I had the energy and drive to do many photo shoots and go on endless auditions. My "manic" energy was actually a plus in New York, and it started to come together for me because I would never give up, no matter what. My roommates and I went to amazing parties, and danced until dawn many nights in a row. I met so many interesting people and got to see so many great plays and shows. I did have a hard time balancing relationships and career. But career came first; I wasn't able to let go of my professional aspirations no matter what.

The stimulation of Manhattan made me feel even more creative, and I started writing more songs and then some short stories. Though I was burning the candle at both ends, I tried to maintain the healthy concepts I'd embraced with my old boyfriend, taking yoga classes and getting involved with Reiki healing. I still went out a lot, though I always kept my drinking to no more than three drinks in an evening. It seemed to work as long as I was careful.

> "I was absolutely determined to have peace and not be controlled by my emotions."

My next serious boyfriend was also a musician. I moved in with him. Just like many other artists, he was having serious financial difficulties. It was while I was with him that the flaming ends of my candle started to burn a little too close to my core. The insecurity caused by his money worries combined with my overdriven life triggered the first manic episode I'd had in a long, long time. I had to move in with a friend in the East Village, and for a while it looked like I might have to give up my ambitions and move back home. I was heartbroken.

But I'd learned something from my spiritual work, and from the experience of making my way in the big city: you have to face your problems. So I saw a doctor, even though it seemed like a step backwards for me. Under his care I stabilized rapidly, and I'm happy to say I haven't needed medication for a very long time. I ended up living in my own place in the East Village for five years and enjoyed every moment of it, making a career for myself in New York just like I'd dreamed of doing.

Living alone gave me the opportunity to focus on healing my mind. I was absolutely determined to have peace and not be controlled by my emotions. I studied a Course in Miracles. I went to yoga and wrote a lot. I learned to feel the pain and resolve my issues in the moment, so that I could keep more negativity from swirling into the grey area of confused emotions.

I still have a musical man in my life, although there is much more balance to this relationship than in any other I have had. He inspires me to continue to be creative and to keep moving forward. I find that as long as I have a project to work on, whether it's producing, writing or acting, I can continue to transform the darkness into light. Having bipolar disorder is very difficult, but I'm proud that I've learned to manage it by facing it. I now understand that even if I get a negative thought or emotion, I can take a step back and realize that it's not going to overtake me or control me. Now, when I hear messages in the music, I don't let them speak to me—I let them speak through me by writing them down.

Sherry Stearn has worked in the entertainment industry for 23 years as a model/spokesperson, actor, lyricist, writer of short stories and screenplays and as the producer of three short films. She also donates her time to the Break the Silence Foundation, a non-profit organization helping young people discover their talents and plan for the future. She is inspired by her collaborations with creative people and finds fulfillment by expressing herself through writing and the arts.

Dear Valerie

Beth Friedlander

Dear Valerie,

It's so great that we found each other after all these years. See, the internet is good for something after all! I'm sorry to hear that you and Steve didn't make it; I hope the divorce didn't hit your children too hard. Be sure to bring lots of pictures to the class reunion. You know, the kind on paper, like we used to have "back in the day."

Things haven't been rosey for Don and me over the years, either, but we're blessed with a good enough relationship to have weathered the storms. Val, we've had some *serious* storms, too. I may as well tell you, because it feels good to get it off my chest, but I was diagnosed bipolar. Back when we were in high school, we called it manic depression. You may remember I told you that my grandmother committed suicide. She was bipolar. My uncle is too. Runs in families. Big time. More on that later.

Where to start? It's hard to explain one's thinking, especially from so long ago, and even more so when that thinking was confused. I'm coming off a long depression right now—at least my family and I pray I'm coming off it. My doctor has started me on a new medication, and it fatigues me so much that I might just go face down on the keyboard; if so, I'll try to hit "Send" on my way down. It can take a while for any medication to kick in. I'm hoping, praying, that this one will work, and soon. I need it to work, Val.

Before I was diagnosed BP, I was in standard therapy for seven years with a psychoanalyst (you know, the whole bit with the couch and everything). When I entered graduate school, he suggested that I work with an analyst in-training, since he thought I needed it, that it would be interesting for a psych student, and because it would enable me to get the treatment very inexpensively. The experience was often boring and seemed to serve little purpose at first, but problems eventually livened it up. You are supposed to have analysis at the end of the day, so you can dream about the issues that come up. Because my classes were at night, my sessions needed to be earlier, which meant that any stirred up material had to be dealt with during the day, while I was very busy with graduate school. Unhappy early experiences did arise during these sessions, and it became more and more difficult to set them aside and concentrate on my studies.

I told my analyst that I was having trouble in school, which then quickly became trouble in life in general: organizing things, getting along with roommates, etc. The next week I told him I was about to have a nervous breakdown. He was really unsympathetic, as if he didn't take me seriously at all. Why be a doctor if you're not going to take your patients' complaints seriously? Within the week I had a full blown break of psychotic thinking. I was not diagnosed bipolar at that point, and since I was in such a state of confusion, I don't even remember what they said about it.

I was also dealing with a love affair that meant everything to me at the time. My boyfriend was a psych grad student in Ohio; I'm sure I told you about Hank. I'd say I meant about a third as much to him as he did to me, and I was always anxious about the relationship. All of my trouble in analysis came around the Christmas holidays, when Hank had come home from school. When he left to go back to school I couldn't handle it at all. I totally broke down and ended up in the hospital for several days.

Eventually I went off to school with him. We lasted about two semesters together. Then, with the strain of school and the dissolving relationship, I fell apart again. I had imagined we were getting married, which of course was what I wanted, even though he had made it pretty clear that it wasn't to be. Still no BP diagnosis. To others I'm sure I was just "crazy." What a terrible feeling, to know others are throwing such a harsh judgment on you, as if people with BP are choosing their behaviors.

> "It's truly a medical miracle. May it last for a good fifty or sixty years!"

With each of these breaks, severe depression would follow. The first only lasted about five weeks. The second was much more severe and lasted possibly nine months. People who haven't experienced actual depression can't imagine how debilitating it is. I was hopeless, helpless. The depression just kept going, so the doctors tried lithium. It worked like a charm within days, much sooner than expected. It was from the success of the lithium that the diagnosis of bipolar disorder finally came.

Val, reviewing all this is an intense and exhausting experience. It reminds me just how disabled I was and still am. I just got this new computer, so rather than break it by passing out on it, that's all for now.

Love,

Beth

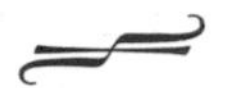

Hi Val,

Thanks for your email. It helps so much that you understand and are willing to listen. It's so oppressive to feel like you're completely alone in your own mind. I have a little more energy and motivation today. I don't want to get my hopes up too high about these new meds, but I can't help it. Fingers crossed.

You asked how Don has handled all of this. While it hasn't been easy by any means, we were blessed with a 20-year "window" where I had, probably, no manifestations of my BP. I was in remission, I was told. So it didn't interfere with our raising Patrick and Diana. Don has been a real rock for me, though it's been hard for him sometimes. I once asked him why he didn't just leave and find someone else. His reply was, "Don't worry about that, I'm not going anywhere. If you want to worry about something, worry about lightning striking."

It's helped that I don't have some of the typical bipolar incidents where I come home with huge purchases or stay out all night. In fact, my manic feelings are more likely to manifest themselves inwardly: I'll get caught up in my own delusional thoughts and feelings privately, while others might not be aware that I am thinking strangely, except to notice that I'm not living up to my responsibilities. I need to stress that being manic from BP—to me, at least—doesn't feel horrible. In fact, it's like being high all (*all*) the time. And, like when someone is high, it's what happens while "under the influence" that can be horrible. Sometimes, though, I just get "silly" (and Don would probably welcome some harmless silliness now, as you will read.)

That 20-year window came crashing shut a few years ago, when I had a very long manic episode. Because of the inward nature of my mania, no one guessed, including Don or my current therapist, that I was having a problem. I did my best to get the therapist to help me, but I simply wasn't heard. I was working at the library and was having trouble concentrating, so I asked my doctor for some medication to help. Nothing untoward happened until a month or so later when the family and I went to a church conference. I started to laugh for no reason. I remember sitting in my room by myself, laughing about anything and everything. It went from silly to embarrassing to dangerous. In the following six months it escalated into a horrendous, sad episode.

Once during this episode, I developed the delusion that my previous therapist had died of cancer, and I made a big donation in his name to the American Cancer Society! I have been told by a subsequent therapist that it was probably my way of emotionally separating from my old therapist when I was already having difficulty with reality.

After that, I plunged into a hellish depression that has lasted now for about four years. If it weren't for this new medication, Val, I wouldn't even be able to move myself to write about it. My days start with very painful mornings, when taking showers seems like running a marathon. Until lately, I have spent much of my mornings on the couch. Later, I miserably struggle through some activity like grocery shopping or doing some chores. TV doesn't do too much for me. I watch Oprah occasionally. I sometimes listen to books on tape or to NPR—if the topic isn't depressing. At times, I have a lot of trouble reading. I take care of my dogs (with difficulty), which are godsends because they get me out of the house. I have done some volunteer work, but I'm never comfortable socially when I'm so depressed. It's frustrating, because I very much want to make a contribution, so I keep trying. Just recently the computer has become a pleasant pastime, as I am sure you can see.

But I have good times, too. They are almost always in the evening, such as when we had dinner with some friends and family in NYC. Don coming home from work brightens my life to no end. I almost always feel better seeing my Patrick and Diana. Occasional lunch with a friend will lift me right out of depression, temporarily. Also, I have a wonderful new therapist who used to be Buddhist, then became a priest. He's wonderful, and I can already see him as my guide. And I need that. Bipolar can make you feel so adrift.

It's possible this makes it sound more tolerable than it is. It's hard even to think about it. But writing this for you is cathartic. I couldn't write this for someone who didn't care about our family. Each one of us has suffered a lot in his/her own way. It's taken a lot of love for us be together still.

Valerie, I hope the new meds work. It would be great to see you and everybody at the reunion, but I have to be able to get there. And I want to have my act together if I do.

Love always,

Beth

Valerie!!!

Great news! I am having a very fine day, because my new medication is working and I haven't been depressed since last Wednesday or so. It's truly a medical miracle. May it last for a good fifty or sixty years! I should mention that the medicines are so much better than they were years ago, and I am watched like a hawk by my doctor and therapist so they can head any craziness off at the pass. People's attitudes towards mental illness and the medical treatments available, have come a long way since we were in high school.

I know I've been very lucky. It's amazing that before the last episode, I'd been given 20 years without trouble. It's enough to make someone believe in God, since I always prayed for enough time to get the kids raised without problems.

Before I get ahead of myself celebrating, let me say that I am worried about Diana. She's had depression and anxiety and we're pretty sure she has BP too. She's being very brave about the whole thing, though; maybe having seen what BP did to me is making her that much more open to treatment options. I told her that I was letting you in on my "family secret" and she thought it was really "cool!" She said if more people talked about this stuff, more people would understand it, and it wouldn't be so bad any more. She's so right. Just sharing this with you has taken such a weight off my heart.

I hope they have non-alcoholic punch at the reunion, because I don't want it to interfere with my medication when I drink a toast to lightning not striking.

Don't forget to bring pictures to the reunion!

Love,

Beth

Beth Friedlander lives in Baltimore, Maryland with her husband and two dogs, and recently purchased a horse. She volunteers in the area of art therapy.

Pushing Forward

Amy Pilkington

After the birth of my third child, I became suicidal. I was diagnosed with postpartum depression and my doctor prescribed an antidepressant. It seemed to be working for a while, but my symptoms eventually got worse and I became suicidal again. I was prescribed another antidepressant and sent for a psychological evaluation to determine if hospitalization was needed. It was a vicious cycle that went on for several years. The symptoms would always subside but then they'd come back with a vengeance. When I was finally diagnosed with bipolar disorder, my initial reaction was a feeling of relief. I assumed that I would start taking medication and that would be the end of it. After my first psychotic break though, I realized that this was far from the truth.

Psychosis was unlike anything I had ever imagined. I thought I was crazy and would have to be institutionalized for the rest of my life. It was the ultimate betrayal of the mind. Trying to figure out what was real and what was imagined proved to be an impossible feat. The hallucinations seemed so real that I completely lost touch with reality. I began hearing voices and having lengthy conversations with imaginary people. My life became a series of events conjured up by my mind. I was afraid that I would be committed and this fear kept me from saying anything to my doctor.

Shortly after my father's death, the hallucinations got much worse. I called my husband at work and told him that I intended to take several bottles of pills. He called the police and they came to my home and stayed with me until my husband arrived. With this suicide attempt thwarted, I was forced to deal with my illness. The doctor strongly recommended hospitalization, but I adamantly refused. I was allowed to go home after my husband assured him that I would remain under constant supervision. I underwent another psychiatric evaluation and I was diagnosed with Bipolar I with psychotic features.

That was the first of several psychotic episodes. I didn't understand why I kept having hallucinations, even though I had been taking my medication as prescribed. After I became suicidal again, I was sent to a private mental hospital for evaluation. Fortunately, they decided not to admit me. It was then that I realized that medication wasn't enough, but I didn't know what more I could do. I came to the conclusion that I would either live out my life in misery or I would eventually commit suicide.

I knew that I couldn't bear this for several more decades, so I had to find a solution before I ended up taking my own life. My husband insisted that I begin attending therapy sessions on a regular basis. I had seen a therapist several times in the past and the results didn't impress me. I reluctantly agreed, and am now thankful that I did. Therapy helped me to understand how I could help myself. My therapist encouraged me to explore my feelings, and he commended me for my efforts. For the first time in several years, I began to have a positive attitude and committed myself to recovery.

During periods of stabilization, I focused on understanding how my illness impacted my family and friends. I realized that it was a struggle for them as well. Relationships are difficult for both sides and dealing with something as difficult as bipolar disorder can cause a great deal of resentment. My husband resented the fact that I was no longer the person he married. I resented him because he didn't understand what I was going through. It's almost as if I have several personalities and he never knows which one he is going to be dealing with. It took me a long time to realize this, but I knew I had to try to make things easier for both of us to save our marriage. It motivated me to push harder.

I began charting my moods and finding small things that affected how I felt. I began to analyze situations that led to rage and tried to learn how I could regain control. In doing so, I improved my self-esteem and I started to feel like I had some control over my life again.

Taking these small steps has greatly improved my quality of life. It certainly isn't a cure and it doesn't prevent episodes, but it has made the episodes less severe and less frequent. In the past six months, I have not had a psychotic, major depressive or full-blown manic episode. I have had a few minor issues with depression and anger, but it has not gotten out of control. The difference has been tremendous and it is something I can live with.

It's important to me to maintain a sense of humor. Setbacks will occur. For me, the hardest part was learning to accept that I can't prevent episodes nor maintain complete control over my actions and emotions. Knowing that it isn't my fault, and that I am putting forth a great deal of effort to do my very best, makes me feel much better about my illness and myself. I no longer feel guilty because I know how hard I work to achieve stability, and that is all that anyone can expect of me. Learning to laugh at myself keeps me from feeling as if every minor setback is a personal failure. If I dwell on it, it is sure to throw me into a depressive episode and I want to avoid that if at all possible.

The support of family and friends is crucial. My family is learning to accept the frequent mood changes associated with my illness. They will jokingly tell others to be careful not to make me mad and they will giggle when I do get upset. If an issue arises that they cannot resolve, they will often ask me to take care of it. I can end a squabble or settle a disagreement faster than anyone. Most people will walk away just because they know they won't win the argument. It's nice to feel needed and useful, even if it is only for conflict resolution. It also allows me to vent my frustrations.

I have also found distractions that help me to remove myself from situations before they get out of hand. It's not unusual to see me carrying around a camera and snapping photos of anything I find interesting. Seeing things through a lens sometimes makes me feel like I am on the outside looking in rather than being in the middle of things. You might catch me fiddling with the plastic zipper pull on my jacket or constantly shaking my leg to get rid of nervous energy. It all sounds silly, but it helps me get through the day.

"Knowing that it isn't my fault... makes me feel much better about my illness and myself."

My goal in life has always been to make a lasting impact on the world. I actively seek out others suffering from bipolar disorder and try to help them understand that they are not alone. I am very open about my illness and happily share my experiences in order to illustrate the day to day struggles. If my efforts can save the life of just one person or prove to someone that you can lead a productive life despite having bipolar disorder, then I will feel as if I have fulfilled my goal.

My doctor continues to monitor me closely for any changes. Until recently, he held my prescriptions in the office and had my husband pick them up. I still struggle with the symptoms of bipolar disorder, but I am determined to keep pushing forward. It will not get the best of me. I may have bipolar disorder, but I don't let it define me.

Don't let it define you.

Amy Pilkington is a freelance writer who is committed to learning to live with bipolar disorder.

Love Has No Boundaries

Carrie McCarter

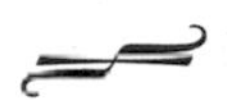

Growing up was hard for me. We were extremely poor and moved regularly. I did not have very nice clothing, and I was skinny. We lived in a bad neighborhood where the kids bullied me, so I had to fight all of the time. By eleventh grade I had been in six high schools. My mother, who was physically, emotionally, and verbally abusive, kicked me out of the house every other week. I never knew my father, but when I got older my mother told me that he had schizophrenia and the last she heard of him, he was in a hospital. When I was 17 years old, I could not take living with my mother anymore, so I moved out.

But my tendency to get into fights got me into trouble, and I eventually joined the Navy. I still had many issues with aggression which led the people in my battalion to say I was crazy. My commander recommended that I go to anger management classes, but after a short time the counselor recommended that I be separated because—though I was not informed of the reason—I had a personality disorder. I was never told of the recommendation, just told I was unfit for sea duty and put on shore duty instead.

While on active duty, I met a man who seemed to accept me for who I was. I ended up pregnant, and after I had the baby, his time in the military was up and I requested release from active duty. I was depressed and was put on medication. But my lack of self control and the sad history with relationships took a toll on my current relationship.

I became a fulltime student and had a second child, and things seemed to get worse. I was diagnosed with postpartum depression and the doctors changed my medication. My husband and I moved to another state, hoping the change would make things better. But things got so bad between us that I almost left him. I didn't and instead became pregnant again. One day, when I was three months pregnant, we argued and I downed a bottle of pills. I was taken to the hospital, and thank God the pills I took did not harm the baby.

"It's a wonderful feeling—the knowledge that my life was worth saving."

I was blessed with a husband who would not give up. By this time, he was constantly searching the internet for explanations for my extreme behavior. He stumbled upon bipolar disorder, and I told my therapist and doctor about it. The doctors started me on Lamictal and Zoloft. But I then had an extreme case of mania, like I'd never experienced before, and chopped off all of my hair. The doctor added Geodon. A few months later I had an argument with a coworker and was reprimanded. Lithium was then added to my cocktail.

Ironically, it was not long after these events that my mother was diagnosed with bipolar disorder. This went some way towards explaining a lot of the turmoil in my past, as well as extra confirmation of my own diagnosis. It took some time for my doctors to adjust the recipe for my cocktail, but we made great progress and I slowly came out of the dark times.

Overall things are a lot better now. I managed to complete my MBA while working full time and spending time with my three children. I am so thankful that my husband thought to search the net; that he cared enough to stick it out and find out what my problem was. That foundation of care made all the difference. And I am thankful to my doctor, who through trials and tribulations finally found the right cocktail with the right dosages. It's a wonderful feeling—the knowledge that my life was worth saving.

Carrie McCarter is a wife and a mother of three. She holds a Bachelor of Arts degree in business management and a Masters degree in business administration in accounting and is currently a corporate manager. She loves traveling, reading and trying new and interesting things.

Resources

On the following pages you will find information on some of the foremost organizations focused on bipolar disorder research, treatment and support.

National and International Organizations for Information and Support

NAMI (National Alliance on Mental Illness)

NAMI Main office
2107 Wilson Boulevard, Suite 300
Arlington, VA 22201-3042
Main: (703) 524-7600
Fax: (703) 524-9094
Information Helpline: 1 (800) 950-NAMI (6264)
Website: www.nami.org

NAMI is the National Alliance on Mental Illness, the nation's largest grass roots organization for people with mental illnesses and their families. Founded in 1979, NAMI has affiliates in every state and in more than 1,100 local communities across the country. NAMI members and friends work to fulfill their mission by providing support, education, and advocacy.

NIMH (National Institute of Mental Health)

National Institute of Mental Health
Science Writing, Press, and Dissemination Branch
6001 Executive Boulevard, Room 8184, MSC 9663
Bethesda, MD 20892-9663
Phone: 1-866-615-6464 (toll-free)

1-866-415-8051 (TTY toll-free)
Fax: (301) 443-4279
Website: www.nimh.nih.gov

NIMH supports more than 2,000 research grants and contracts at universities and other institutions across the country and overseas. Investigators propose projects themselves through grant applications and must apply for renewals at intervals in order to receive continued funding.

NARSAD (National Alliance for Research on Schizophrenia and Depression)
60 Cutter Mill Road, Suite 404
Great Neck, NY 11021
Phone: (800) 829-8289 (toll-free)
Fax: (516) 487-6930
Website: www.narsad.org/research

NARSAD supports scientific research to find better treatments and ultimately prevent severe mental illnesses.

DBSA (Depression and Bipolar Support Alliance)
730 N. Franklin Street, Suite 501
Chicago, Illinois 60654-7225
Phone: 1-800-826-3632 (toll-free)
Fax: (312) 642-7243
Website: www.dbsalliance.org

DBSA offers information on depression and bipolar disorder as well as listings to patient support groups across the USA.

Foundation For Mood Disorders
952 Fifth Avenue, Suite 6A
New York, NY 10075
Phone: (212) 772-3400
Fax: (212) 288-0809

Website: www.foundationformooddisorders.com

Foundation for Mood Disorders' goal is to complete a study on the neuro-protective properties of lithium.

ISBD (International Society for Bipolar Disorders)
P.O. Box 7168
Pittsburgh, PA 15213-0168
Phone: (412) 802-6940
Fax: (412) 802-6941
Website: www.isbd.org

The Society aims to foster ongoing international collaboration regarding education and research with an objective to advance the treatment of all aspects of bipolar disorders, resulting in improvements in quality of life for those with bipolar disorders and their significant others.

Mental Health America
2000 N. Beauregard Street, 6th Floor
Alexandria, VA 22311
Phone: (703) 684-7722
Toll free: (800) 969-6642
TTY: (800) 433-5959
Fax: (703) 684-5968
Website: www.mentalhealthamerica.net

Mental Health America (formerly known as the National Mental Health Association) is the country's leading nonprofit organization dedicated to helping all people live mentally healthier lives. The goals of their programs are to educate the public, encourage reform, and promote the use of effective local and regional prevention and recovery programs.

MDF The BiPolar Organisation
Castle Works 21 St. George's Road
London
SE1 6ES
United Kingdom
0845 634 0540 (UK Only)/ 0044 207 793 2600 (Rest of World)
Website: www.mdf.org.uk

MDF The BiPolar Organisation aims to enable people affected by manic depression to take control of their lives through the services that we offer members including self-help groups, information and publications, employment advice, self-management training programme, 24-hour legal advice line for employment, legal, benefits and debt issues.

Child and Adolescent Bipolar Resources

Child and Adolescent Bipolar Foundation
1187 Wilmette Avenue
PMB 331
Wilmette, IL 60091
Phone: (847) 256-8525
Fax: (847) 920-9498
Website: www.bpk.org

A parent-led, not-for-profit, web-based membership organization that includes families raising children diagnosed with, or at risk for, pediatric bipolar disorder.

The Juvenile Bipolar Research Foundation
550 Ridgewood Road
Maplewood, NJ 07040
Phone: 866-333-JBRF (National Toll-Free)
Fax: 973-275-0420
Website: www.bpchildresearch.org
E-mail: info@jbrf.org

The first charitable organization solely dedicated to the support of research for the study of early-onset bipolar disorder.

NYU Child Study Center
577 First Avenue
New York, NY 10016
Phone: (212) 263-6622
Website: www.aboutourkids.org

The NYU Child Study Center was founded in 1997 to improve the treatment of child psychiatric disorders through scientific practice, research, and education and to eliminate the stigma of being or having a child with a psychiatric disorder.

Support for Family Members and Caregivers

GLAXOSMITHKLINE
Phone: (888) 825-5249
Website: www.bipolar.com

Run by a large drug company, this site/ source nonetheless offers valuable information for family and friends of bipolar disorder sufferers.

The Family Center For Bipolar Disorder
Ms. Annie Steele, FC for BD Program Coordinator
Department of Psychiatry
Beth Israel Medical Center
New York, NY 10003
Phone: (212) 420-2204
Website: www.bpfamily.org

The Family Center involves the families of bipolar patients at every stage of care. The program is dedicated to improving patients' outcome and quality of life, and also protecting family members—including children—from the pain, frustration, isolation, and misunderstanding that are the norm.

NNAAMI (National Network of Adult and Adolescent Children who have a Mentally Ill Parent)
Mr. Paul Mckillop, Convenor
P.O. Box. 213
Glen Iris. 3146
Melbourne, Victoria. Australia
Phone / Fax +61 3 98893095

Children breaking the silence, we are a group of people who have experienced life with a mentally ill parent. We established NNAAMI to provide assistance for one another, via self-help support, discussion groups and counseling.

Top Bipolar Research, Diagnostic and Clinical Care Institutions

Massachusetts General Hospital Bipolar Clinic and Research Program
Gary Sachs, Founder and Director
50 Staniford Street Suite 580
Boston, MA 02114
Phone: (617) 726-6188
(617) 726-5855 (for clinical care appointments)
Website: www.manicdepressive.org

This program is dedicated to providing quality clinical care, conducting clinically informative research, and educating colleagues and patients, as well as the greater community about bipolar disorder.

Johns Hopkins Mood Disorders Program
Department of Psychiatry and Behavioral Science
600 North Wolfe Street
Baltimore, MD 21287-7413
Phone: (410) 955-3130
Fax: (410) 955-0946

Website: www.hopkinsmedicine.org/psychiatry/moods

The expert psychiatric faculty at Johns Hopkins studies mood disorders from all perspectives and is committed to educating other health professionals and the general public about these illnesses.

UCLA Mood Disorders Clinic/Research Program
Dr. Lori Altshuler, Director of UCLA
Mood Disorders Research Program
Dr. Michael Gitlin, Director of Mood Disorders Clinic
300 UCLA Medical Plaza Suite 1544
Los Angeles, CA 90095
Phone: (310) 794-MOOD (6663)
Website: www.semel.ucla.edu/mood

The UCLA Mood Disorders Research Program (MDRP) focuses on exploring the etiology of mood disorders through neuroimaging, evaluating factors associated with vulnerability to mood episodes, and finding new treatment options for individuals suffering from mood disorders.

Case Western University
Bipolar Disorder Research Center
Co-Director Dr. Joseph Calabrese
Office Phone: 216-844-2865
W.O. Walker Center
10524 Euclid Avenue
Cleveland, Ohio
Office Fax: 216-844-2875
Appointment Phone: 216-844-2850

This research center believes in a "team approach," as it employs clinicians with diverse skills and credentials. They work together to provide balanced care, with an equal emphasis on medications and psychological therapy.

Columbia University Psychiatry
Columbia University Medical Center
622 West 168th Street
New York, NY 10032
Phone: (212) 305-600
Website: columbiapsychiatry.org

Columbia Psychiatry offers levels of care including complete evaluation, inpatient and intensive outpatient treatment for mood disorders including bipolar disorder. Also offers a referral line and family therapy.

Stanford School of Medicine Bipolar Disorders Clinic
Clinic Chief Terence A. Ketter, M.D.
401 Quarry Road
Stanford, CA 94305-5723
Phone: (650) 724-4795
Website: http://bipolar.stanford.edu/

The Bipolar Disorders Clinic is part of the Department of Psychiatry and Behavioral Sciences at Stanford University School of Medicine. It offers on-going clinical treatment, manages clinical trials and neuroimaging studies, provides lectures, and teaches seminar courses at Stanford University and trains residents in the School of Medicine.

The Stanley Medical Research Institute
E. Fuller Torrey, M.D., Executive Director
8401 Connecticut Avenue Suite 200
Chevy Chase, MD 20815
Phone: (301) 571-0760
Fax: (301) 571-0769
Website: www.stanleyresearch.org/dnn
Website: www.semel.ucla.edu/mood/research

The Stanley Medical Research Institute (SMRI) is a nonprofit organization supporting research on the causes of, and treatments for, schizophrenia and bipolar disorder. Since it began in 1989, SMRI has supported more than $300 million in research in over 30 countries around the world.

Legal Advice—Rights Regarding Medical Insurance and Disability

Mental Health Benefits Project

Executive Director Wendy Brennan
Advocacy Associate Becky Pietsch
505 8th Avenue, Suite 1103
New York, NY 10018
Phone: 212.684.3365
Helpline: 212.684.3264
Fax: 212.684.3364

Affiliated with NAMI's New York office (see above), the Project informs consumers of their rights under the law and makes referrals.

Treatment Advocacy Center

E. Fuller Torrey, M.D., Founder of the
Treatment Advocacy Center
200 North Glebe Road Suite 730
Arlington, VA 22203
Phone: (703) 294-6001 & (703) 294-6002
Fax: (703) 294-6010
Website: www.treatmentadvocacycenter.org

The Treatment Advocacy Center promotes laws, policies, and practices for the delivery of psychiatric care and supports the development of innovative treatments for and research into the causes of severe and persistent psychiatric illnesses, such as schizophrenia and bipolar disorder.

Allsup
300 Allsup Place
Belleville, IL 62223
Phone: (800) 854-1418
Fax: (618) 236-5778
Website: www.allsup.com

Allsup is partnered with Social Security Disability Insurance (SSDI), which is a payroll tax-funded, federal insurance program.

Suicide Prevention, Information and Support

The National Suicide Prevention Lifeline
1-800-273-TALK (8255)

AFSP (American Foundation for Suicide Prevention)
120 Wall Street
22nd Floor
New York, NY 10005
Phone: 1-888-333-AFSP (2377)
Fax: (212) 363-6237
Website: www.afsp.org

The American Foundation for Suicide Prevention (AFSP) is the leading national not-for-profit organization exclusively dedicated to understanding and preventing suicide through research, education and advocacy, and to reaching out to people with mental disorders and those impacted by suicide.

The Jason Foundation
181 East Main Street
Jefferson Building, Suite 5
Hendersonville, TN 37075
Website: www.jasonfoundation.com

The Jason Foundation, Inc. is dedicated to the prevention of the "Silent Epidemic" of youth suicide through educational and awareness programs to equip young people, educators/youth workers, and parents with the tools and resources to help identify and assist at-risk youth.

Yellow Ribbon Suicide Prevention Program
PO Box 644
Westminster, CO 80036-0644
Phone: (303) 429-3530
Fax: (303) 426-4496
Website: www.yellowribbon.org

Yellow Ribbon is a community-based program that empowers and educates through seminars and support groups. This is a program of "people helping people." Donations are received from supporters within these communities.

The Jed Foundation
Courtney Knowles, Executive Director
220 Fifth Avenue 9th Floor
New York, NY 10001
Phone: (212) 647-7544
Fax: (212) 647-7542
Website: www.jedfoundation.org

As the nation's leading organization working to reduce emotional distress and prevent suicide among college students, The Jed Foundation is protecting the mental health of students across the country.

The Karla Smith Foundation
10101 West Main Street
Belleville, IL 62223
Phone: (888) KSF-HOPE
Website: www.karlasmithfoundation.org

Karla Smith's seven-year struggle with bipolar disorder began when she was 19. It culminated with her suicide at age 26. Karla

Smith Foundation, founded by Tom, her father, Fran, her mother, and Kevin, her twin brother, is an avenue to share family experiences which similarly impact thousands of others.

Send Us Your Story

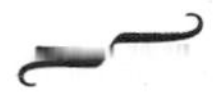

Do you have a story to tell? LaChance Publishing and The Healing Project publish stories written by people like you. Have you or those you know been touched by life-threatening illness or chronic disease? Your story can give comfort, courage and strength to others who are going through what you have already faced.

Your story should be no less than 500 words and no more than 2,500 words. You can write about yourself or someone you know. Your story must inform, inspire, or teach others. Tell the story of how you or someone you know faced adversity; what you learned that would be important for others to know; how dealing with the disease strengthened or clarified your relationships or inspired positive changes in your life.

The easiest way to submit your story is to visit the LaChance Publishing website at www.lachancepublishing.com. There you will find guidelines for submitting your story online, or you may write to us at submissions@lachancepublishing.com. We look forward to reading your story!

For the duration of the printing and circulation of this book, for every book that is sold by LaChance Publishing, LaChance will contribute 100% of the net proceeds to The Healing Project, LLC. The Healing Project can be reached at 12 Warren Place, Brooklyn, NY 11217. The Healing Project is dedicated to promoting the health and well being of individuals challenged by life threatening or chronic illness and to developing resources to enhance their quality of life and the lives of their families. The Healing Project is a tax exempt organization as described in Revenue Code Section 501(c) (3).